FEARLESSNESS

Lyanne Truong

This book is dedicated to the men and women whom served in the armed forces. The freedom and liberties that we enjoy are only possible because of their dedication and sacrifices.

Contents

Group V. <u>FEARFUL with RIGID/ATTACHED NOTION</u>

PURPOSE

Working with those who may be dying is part of my everyday job.

And, based on over a decade of treating cancer patients, I have learned that medication is only part of the battle against disease. In most cases, a very important weapon that is needed to successfully fight illness is missing: A new concept of intervention which I call **Fearlessness**.

I have introduced **Fearlessness** to my patients to calm their fright, bring fulfilment to their lives and often, free them from their disease.

The progression of their disease can be **delayed**, and some even **reversed** with implementation of **Fearlessness.**

INTRODUCTION

Why do some patients' treatments fail and their disease progresses much quicker than for others? For over a decade, this troubling question had repeatedly led me to see a common pattern of problems that not only existed in my deceased patients, but also in those that are being treated.

As you may know, many medical experts, researchers, and pharmaceutical companies invested years of their time and millions of dollars in hopes of developing better and improved medications to treat diseases including the advanced stages of cancers. Often, their hard work was unfairly rewarded because diseases remained unimproved and the survival rate of cancer patient was only extended for a short period of time.

Initially, my approach was actually similar to theirs; to provide and find the best medication to fight diseases. But as time continued, a common problem emerged from extensive observation of treating cancer patients.

The direct contact and observation of treating cancer patients had ascertained me to predict which patients would be able to tolerate treatment and delay the progression of the disease. The breakthrough of **Fearlessness** concept of intervention became so crucial that it laid new ground for me to practice medicine.

What is **Fearlessness** and why is **Fearlessness** necessary?

Fearlessness is a process initially designed to help the cancer patient deal with difficult emotional experiences that they go through from the time they are diagnosed with cancer.

A diagnosis of cancer is rightfully scary to anyone who receives it from their health care provider. The typical patient deals with it similarly to the way they deal with loss. The patient and their family often go through a denial process. They become upset and angry that cancer happened to them. They seek a second opinion to assure that they do indeed have cancer and that treatment is necessary and is appropriate. At times, they blame the previous provider if the disease continues to progress. Some become depressed especially when the treatment fails. Few even turn against their faith.

Fearlessness does not involve the use of pharmaceuticals and is a vital weapon that is needed to successfully fight illness.

The following anecdotal evidences are of my patients who have been introduced to this concept of **Fearlessness**.

Group I

FEARFUL UNKNOWN FUTURE

Chapter 1

Malaise

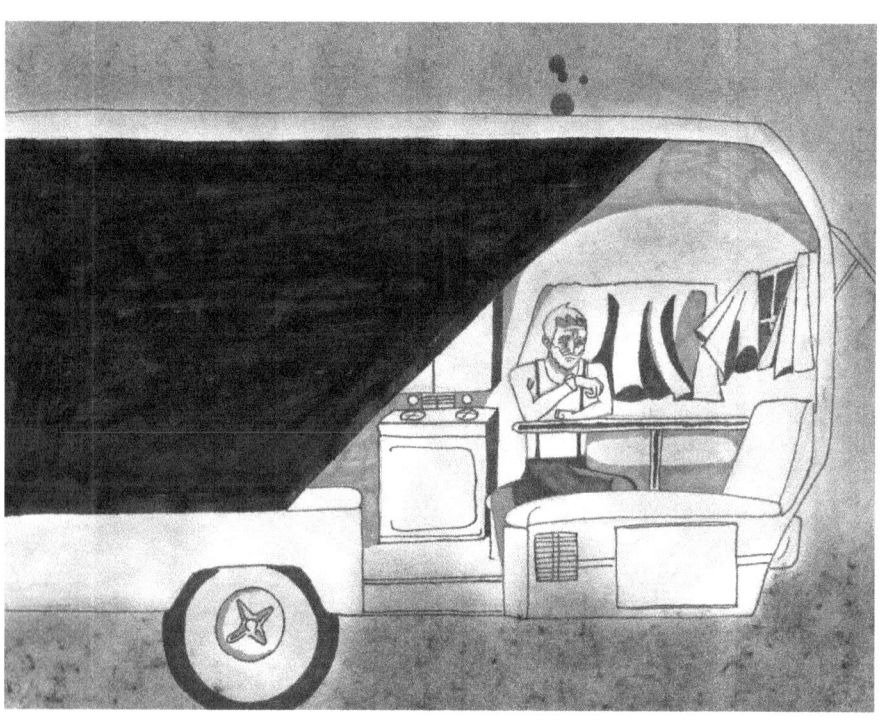

Mr. Carl Colorado is an elderly patient who has a long list of medical diseases. Over a period of five years, he had gone through all the standard treatments for Idiopathic/immune thrombocytopenia purpura (ITP) including laparoscopic splenectomy to remove his spleen. He had received about 10 different treatments including the newest medication that was just released by the FDA for ITP. However, his diseases continued to worsen. He coded (near death) and hospitalized many times and requiring very close observation.

During his visitations, he was **very restless**, **anxious** and especially **impatient,** and always complained of **tiredness**. He expressed **fear** and **doubt** about the newly increased doses of his medication. His blood counts persisted on a downward trend while on the newest medication. I perceived the new medication was going to fail, since his disease was heading toward a critical point.

After noting his lack of progress with no new medication available, I tried a new and different approach; the concept of **Fearlessness**. I was set to search for other causes to his disease**.** During this time, I recalled wondering how he was capable of worrying as much as he did. His worries were about everything and anything, non-stop. He was up all night, or barely slept because he worried he would oversleep and would miss my appointment (or any appointment for that matter). He watched the clock very closely so he would not miss his medications. He was on so many medications that he felt he could open a small pharmacy. He constantly worried about his illnesses and his grandson's well-being. Whenever he was awake, his time was spent inside his house. His only entertainment was listening to religious talk shows, or worrying about the next hour, and his grandson who once mocked him. He was worrying and stressing over **the fear of the unknown future!**

As the searching proceeded, he revealed the trouble of his only son named River, who had a long history of drug addiction and jail time. When River's wife left him, Mr. Colorado helped raise his two young boys. River and his two boys moved in with Mr. Colorado in his small mobile home. For years, Mr. Colorado continued to help his son and hoped he would change and clean up his act. Mr. Colorado raised the two boys while River was in and out of drugs or jail time. At the time, one of the grandsons died in a car accident before he turned twenty three years of age.

After receiving a death beneficiary of forty two thousand dollars, River, because of his addictions, spent all of the money in three months. Mr. Colorado continued to tolerate with River's abuse until he turned eighty years old. With help from his second grandson, he sought a restraining order to keep River away from the mobile home preventing any more stealing. Mr.

Colorado however, continued to worry about his son's health, and actually wanted to let him back into the house. His only surviving grandson became very precious.

Mr. Colorado constantly worried about his grandson who is in his early twenties and still resided with him. His worries turned into an overly protective and vigilant part of his daily routine. He distrusted the grandson's girlfriend. He thought she was not sincere and a bad influence. He felt she was only after his money and a place to stay. He concluded that she would leave his grandson as soon as inheritance was received. Mr. Colorado had planned to leave him the old mobile home wishing he had more to give. During that moment, I couldn't help thinking about his mobile home's condition. I recalled a winter visit when he came to see me, wearing a paper thin jacket and obviously hungry.

I found out he did not have much to eat and could not fix his meals. The stove was malfunctioning and had been for several years. To operate the stove, he would have to use pliers to turn it on and off. He stressed over the fact that his grandson would suffer enduring great misery, predicting that the girlfriend would take off with his money. He knew that the grandson loved her dearly, but incapable of seeing the other side of her and stressed over that thought. He hoped he could tell his grandson gently without getting into a fight.

I spent several months working with him, explaining that his grandson, now a grown man, should make his own decisions and take responsible for his actions. He struggled unable to let go of his worries and fears about his grandson's future.

I was unable to help him see this for many more months, but as quickly as he realized that he did not have any control over his grandson's life nor future, he started to change. He became calmer and more patient. His blood pressure was under control. He was happier and started to spend more time outside the house. He went to the doughnut shop near his house. He stayed at the doughnut shop for coffee and played chess several times a day. His platelet levels became more stable and his treatment started to work. The treatment began to work better. The frequency of treatments was extended longer and longer. His visits became less and less. He eventually came off of ITP treatment and was placed on observation. The need to restart treatment for his blood disease was delayed. Occupied with other and new activities in his daily life, his blood disease continued to show good response without any treatment for over a year. He missed a couple follow up visits here and there during which time the blood counts would trend down a bit, but quickly returned to normal range as he focused on himself and not his grandson. He was doing well, but started missing more appointments.

Over a five month period with several appointment reminders, he did not show up for follow up. Suddenly, Mr. Colorado was brought to the emergency department by his grandson for sudden onset of altered mental status and was admitted to the hospital.   During the hospital stay, he had a neurological work up to evaluate his sudden change of mental stability. He was found to have a brain tumor located in the center of his brain.   As it turned out, Mr. Colorado's closest sister had been ill for several months and passed away two weeks prior to this onset of his mental instability. For months, he was constantly worrying about her illness and her passing. This was quickly followed by his mental instability as the grandson related later when he came by to inform me of his grandfather's unfortunate news. The neurosurgeon had identified that the brain tumor was very dangerous for biopsy hence, his grandson decided to transfer Mr. Colorado to palliative care for comfort care.   He remained there seven weeks prior to his passing.

Discussion 1:
In this first story, Mr. Colorado lived his life endlessly with worry and fear. He worried and stressed over the **fear of the unknown future**. As you can see, Mr. Colorado was frequently up all night barely sleeping. He watched his clock very closely spending most of his valuable time inside his house. These behaviours are the results of fear.   What caused Mr. Colorado's fear? He yearns for his troubled son to change and wanting

to provide protection so that his only surviving grandson would not suffer. Mr. Colorado spent his time worrying about the next hour. Therefore, he was always very restless, anxious, impatient, fatigued, tired, fearful and doubtful. As soon as he accepted that he had no control over what will happen in the future, he started to adjust his life. He occupied his daily life with new activities.   Instead of spending all his time at home, he left the house and visited the doughnut shop for coffee and played chess several times a day. Losing his closest sister restarted the process of **fear**.

Words to live by

Philippians 4:7:
And the peace of God, which passeth all understanding, shall keep your hearts and minds through Christ Jesus.

Chapter 2
Nervousness

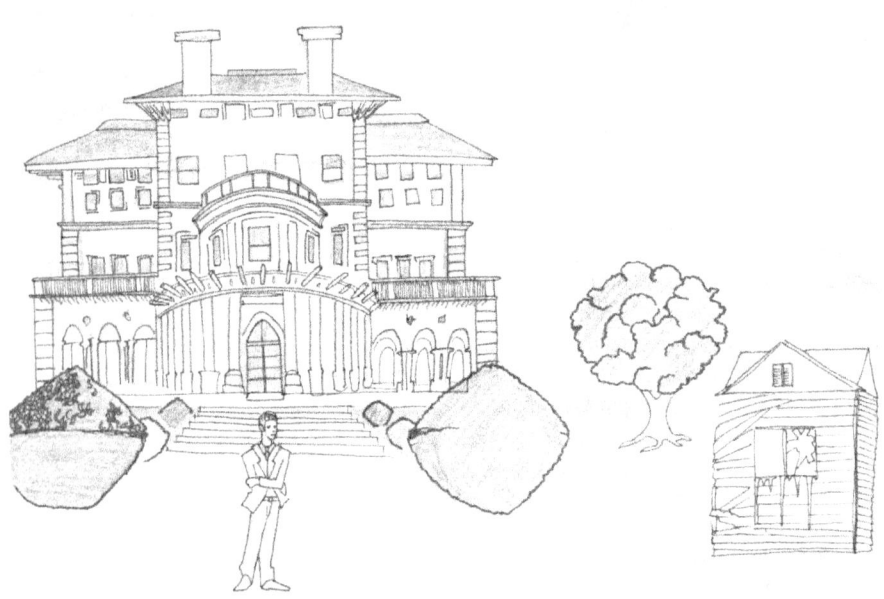

Mr. Harry Hawaii is a patient with few past medical problems, most likely due to his busy life style. His blood counts were found abnormal. He was referred to evaluate for his low blood counts. These low blood counts were known as pancytopenia. Mr. Hawaii was a pleasant, calm individual, but nervous when speaking about his family. In the past, he had abused recreational drugs and liquor. He claimed to have heavily abused drugs for only two years, but continued to drink socially with his clients as well as with his friends.

Due to his pancytopenia, he was recommended to have a bone marrow biopsy. The result revealed that he had a disease known as myelodysplasic syndrome (MDS) and immune thrombocytopenia purpura (ITP).

After learning of the diagnosis, he became more anxious not from the diagnosis, but rather from some unsettling issues. He was introduced to the concept of **Fearlessness** in search of the cause of his fear and to reduce his **anxiety** and **nervousness**. After several months of searching to resolve his fear, he began to open up. He revealed that he was a high earning individual who was struggling with finances over the last five months. He had lost his business. He feared that his family and their wealthy life style would suffer and they would have a difficult time coping. They lived in a large beautiful house and owned several nice cars. His wife hadn't worked since he started the business over fifteen years ago.

At each visitation, he would disclose a little more about his worries exposing a somewhat untrusting and protective character. His blood work would fluctuate up and down depending on how stressful and worried he was. This fluctuation continued for a year. When the blood counts did not fluctuate back up, we revisited the concept of **Fearlessness** to continue the search.

After several more months, his distrusting and protective traits weakened and he began to acknowledge his fear. Now, he unveiled the most dreadful fear frustrating him for the past year. His ex-partner who was his mentor and a very close friend of the family continued to press for payments even after they both lost the business. He constantly worried about not having the money to pay his ex-partner. He was living with a **fearful future**!

Without a doubt, we worked extremely hard to mend his **fear**. Recalling this particular session because Mr. Hawaii stated that he hesitated to involve his wife since she never wanted to have anything to do with his business.

Unbelievably, the very next visit, he brought his wife to the clinic. I was shocked and showed he and his wife his blood work results. For the very first time, the downward trending blood work suddenly fluctuated up, reaching the normal range. Looking at the result, he turned to me with a smirk, confessing that he had resolved the haunting issue with his ex-partner two weeks ago. They were able to come to a peaceful agreement and Mr. Hawaii no longer had to pay him.

His blood work continued to remain stable within normal range for nine months. Then his blood work started to fluctuate down again. He again did not, or was unable, to reveal the truth of his **fear**, but rather, complained indirectly. The complaints were of body rashes, painful dried feet, abdominal discomfort, and a hardened tooth plaque that he thought it may be cancer.

I again ordered imaging for his abdominal pain and tests for each of those complaints. The results were all normal. The hardened plaque was removed after teeth cleaning by the dentist. By this time, many weeks of searching had been conducted to reduce his **fear**. He slowly revealed that he was undergoing bankruptcy and was losing everything. He was down to only one car and the family had moved into a much smaller, somewhat run down house. While he was looking for work, his blood levels fluctuated constantly. On one occasion, his blood levels hit bottom when he did not get a position which was certain that he would get. At this time, he was very frightened that if his counts continued to drop further that he would then need to start treatment. He started to work on his worries, stresses and **fear**.

As quickly as he accepted the need to let go of his **fear** related to his finances, he was able to stay focused on the present and simply work to make the best of what he had. After relinquishing these worries and stresses, not surprisingly, his blood work returned to a normal range again. This process took over three years. He finally learned to accept and make peace with his **fear** and worries. He remained focused on the present and started to work harder, working two jobs. His wife also started working part time. He took a second job in a warehouse which was not easy for this once high earning individual.

When he was happy, so was his blood work; it was stable. He continued to do well so his follow ups had been spaced out farther apart as his blood levels continued to remain stable. His life as well as his family started to pick up the pieces. He now worked for a well-known and large corporation and continued to work in the warehouse part time.

I predict that he will be able to remain healthy as long as he continues to apply himself and remain focused on one day at time. He currently is doing well and has not required any further treatment.

Discussion 2:
In this second story, Mr. Hawaii was living in a **fearful future** of fear of the uncertainty. He became anxious and nervous when he spoke of his family. He **feared** that his family and their accustomed wealthy life style would suffer and they would have a difficult time coping due to the loss of his financial success. His greatest fear

was an inability to provide for his family comfortably. His **fear** seemed to be inevitable and it began to consume his life and health. Once he recognized his fear and became aware of his concerns and worries, he began to adjust his life. As soon as he accepted his reality, he was able to overcome his fear. Instead of owning and running another company, he started to work for one. He also took a second job working at a warehouse which was not easy for him since he was once a wealthy individual. His wife who never worked also adjusted and began to work as well. As a result of letting go of his fear, his family was able to pick up the pieces; he began to fulfill their lives and he was able to gain freedom from his disease.

Words to live by

From the Ten Commandments:
10. Thou shall not covet: can be translated to mean do not want more and more.

Chapter 3

Impatience

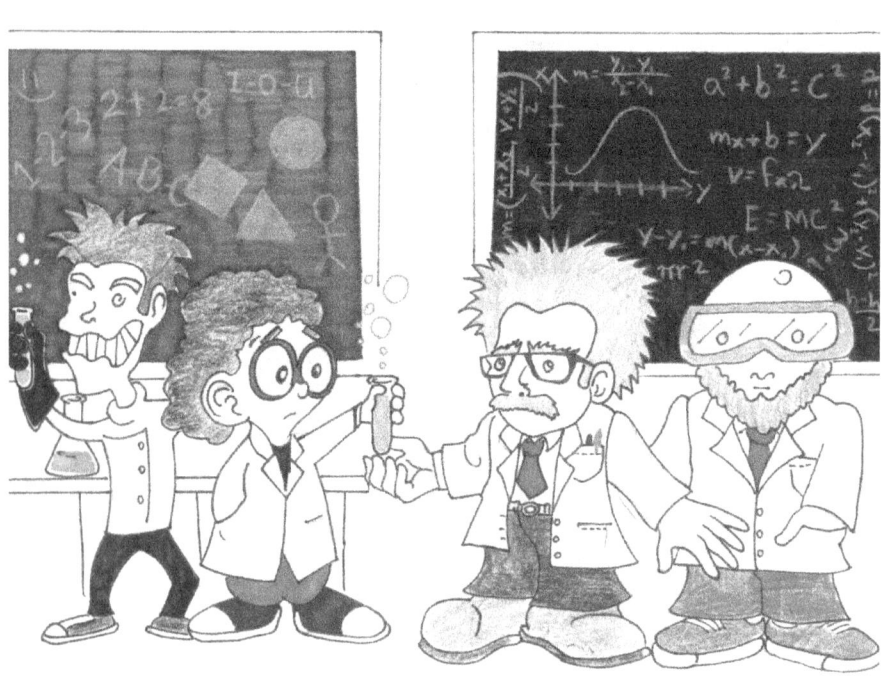

Mr. Mark Montana is an interesting individual, yet a common patient. He is a young patient when compared to most patients with hematological and oncological disease patients. He was referred to evaluate for his low blood counts or pancytopenia.

On his first visit, he showed up late and threatened to leave if he was not seen soon. He was extremely **impatient, erratic** and **combative**. He had a long history of drug abuse and a problematic family. He was in drug rehabilitation at age fourteen. He claimed that he no longer abused heavy street drugs, but only abused alcohol and marijuana on the weekends. His blood counts were severely depressed; a bone marrow biopsy was ordered.

No time was wasted with him and he was introduced to the concept of **Fearlessness** in an effort to identify the source of his **anger.** Unfortunately there are many types of street drugs available and are easy to obtain. Even without resources, addicts can place themselves in danger. It is surprising how quickly, filthy drugs can be "whipped up" from junk to sustain a "high." Cooking up old plastic and toxic waste and using deadly contaminated needles are ways that they waste lives away. Listening to him detail his experience and drug abuse, I could not help but compare drug abusers to pharmaceutical scientists. If pharmaceutical scientists/chemists and drug abusers were in competition, drug abusers could easily defeat them in a race to produce new drugs.

Mr. Montana was not only very interesting, but an extremist. After his first introduction to the **Fearlessness** concept, he quickly converted to a complete vegan. In just one month he stopped drinking alcohol and abusing drugs as well as giving up sodas altogether. After several more months of follow ups, his impatient and erratic behaviour slowly improved, but his **distrust** was difficult to modify. He was very **conflicted** at times. He had trouble accepting his disease. He continually asked why he was not given medications before his symptoms worsened. Unquestionably, he was searching for a cure for his diseases. He was **unhappy**, **unsatisfied** and **doubted** that he was receiving the best treatment since he was not on any medication. He constantly required revisiting the concept of **Fearlessness**.

After several more months, he began to reveal the source of his conflict. For years, he had an enormous animosity toward his physically abusive, alcoholic father, who was never around while he was growing up. He was very angry with his father and blamed him for his drug and alcoholic abuse. His resentment toward his father was so severe that he did not shed a tear during his funeral nor visit his grave since his father's burial over seven years ago. Besides mending his anger with his deceased father, I constantly needed to reiterate that his disease did not require treatments at the time, but that he should be monitored closely. He was persistently seeking answers to cure his diseases. He was living with a **rigid notion** but more so, he was very **fearful of the unknown future!**

After many long hours of repeated sessions of **Fearlessness**, he was able to come to terms with his problems. Beside his father, he later revealed that he also had much resentment and frustration with his mother. He thought she was over powering and controlling. While working on improving relations with his mother, he asked if he could bring her along to his following visits.

On her first visit, she also showed a high degree of impatience, was erratic and controversial. He was a replica of her. She constantly suggested that he seeks second opinions at a well-known cancer institution and was willing to cover part of his bills. She too required introduction to **Fearlessness** for her rigid notion that medication was the solution to cure his illnesses.

Prior to her attending the visit, his blood counts had been fluctuating up and down. His blood counts fluctuated up, remained unchanged for a very short period of time, and then quickly fluctuated back down. The very next visit after her first visit, an amazing surprise occurred with his blood work. The blood counts for the very first time reached normal range. Fortunately, his mother was present again along with his wife and the result was shared with them as well. Unexpectedly, he stated that he made peace with his dead dad at his grave and had a good cry just three days prior to his appointment.

After this visit, his mother started to treat Mr. Montana with more respect and as a grown man. She stopped doubting his judgment. Since then, his patience and blood work have shown improvement.

Even after a year, his blood work remained in the normal range. He constantly works on reducing his stress level of **fear**. He continues to maintain a worry/stress free life style. When it was time for his follow up visits, he modestly stated that he will continue working on reducing his anger. At times, he would wait over an hour to be seen, but waited now patiently and graciously. In the past, he would never be able to do so without becoming anxious, erratic and agitated. He has such a great understanding of the concept of Fearlessness that he has been able to remain happy and easy going. He transformed from an impatient, erratic, conflicted individual, to a very patient, understanding and calm individual. Most interestingly, he stated that he will continue working hard on reducing his stress and temper every day! He continues with his follow ups without any treatment to date.

Discussion 3:
In the beginning of the third story, Mr. Montana was an extremely impatient, erratic, combative, angry, distrustful, conflicted, unhappy and doubtful individual.   Why did Mr. Montana have

these personality traits? Why was he persistently seeking answers to cure his diseases? He was living with a **rigid** notion but more so, very **fearful** of the **unknown future**. His insistence on finding the cure to his disease was the result of his **fear**. But why was he so fearful and angry? Mr. Montana was filled with resentment and frustration from his past. He lived his life constantly searching for answers and trying to resolve the conflict from his problematic childhood and family. The enormous animosity toward his physically abusive and alcoholic father, who was never around as he was growing up, and the resentment and the frustration toward his mother who was over controlling were situations he constantly battled to avoid in his life which led to the anger that was ultimately created by fear. Unable to resolve his fear, he lived his life recklessly. He felt trapped and hence the unhealthy personality traits resulted. How did he resolve his fear? He was willing to accept and let go of his past. He visited his father's grave and had a long cry for the first time. He worked hard to make peace with his over powering and controlling mother, who never stop doubting him. As a result of letting go of his past, he was able to face his reality.

Words to live by

Taoism:
"When you are content to be simply yourself and don't compare or compete, everybody will respect you."

Chapter 4

Anxiety

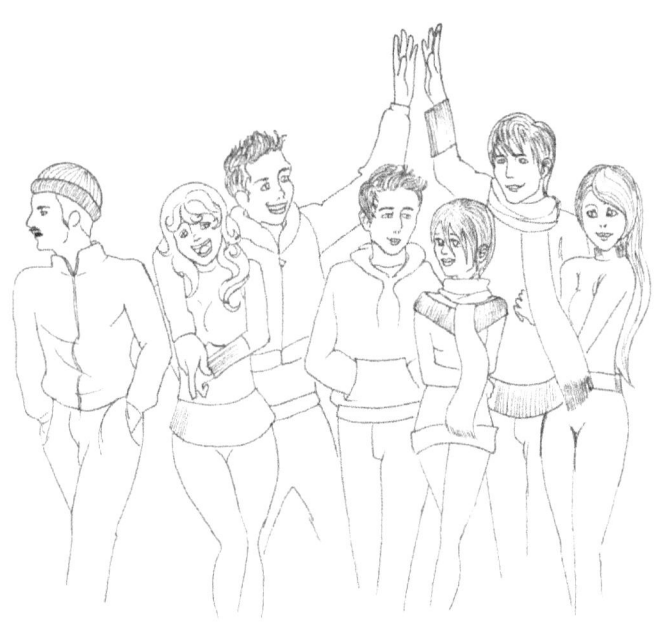

Mr. Dodge Don is a patient, like many of my patients, who has multiple medical problems which include congestive heart failure and hypertension, but was unusual in that he had syphilis at age nineteen. Previously, he had been treated at an infectious disease clinic to insure that he did not have neurosyphillis, aspergillosis, cryptococcus or brucella as an infection that caused his leukocytosis. Fortunately, the results were negative. He was referred to our clinic for his persistent leukocytosis. Erythrocytosis is an abnormally high level of hematocrit and haemoglobin.

When he first came to the clinic, he had multiple complaints of bone pain, general weakness, muscle ache, trouble breathing and the need to open his mouth to breathe. But upon a closer look at him, he was breathing similarly to many of my **anxiety** patients. The opening of his mouth was barely noticeable because his mustache covered his upper lip. He was also so anxious that he was unable to sit for more than three minutes. At the end of his first visit, a Head CT scan was arranged to further evaluate what was thought to be his sinus related problems rather than an infectious process.

At the next visit, he continued to complain of stress and requested that something be done to better his breathing. He claimed to have lost control to close his mouth, and it was due to having to open his mouth in order to breathe. He returned after having his imaging done. We went over the result of the head CT scan which showed that he had mild sinusitis and possible inflammation of the jaw joint. At the end of the visit, he was referred to the ENT (EAR Nose and Throat specialists) and dentist. He quickly arranged to be seen by the dentist who assured him there was no tooth decay or infection in his gum that could cause his jaw joint problem, but thought that he may have a slight dislocation of the jaw joint. The dentist referred him to the Maxillofacial Surgeon for his Temporomandibular joint (TMJ-joint, where the skull and lower jaw meet in front of ear) which he thought was the cause of the slightly dislocated jaw. He was told by the specialist, that if he wished, he could have his jaw surgically repaired.

He saw me on the same day as his dentist visit. On this particular visit, he became extremely anxious and his breathing was at its worst. His blood pressure was also extremely high. Unsurprisingly, his blood work, particularly the white blood count or leukocytosis, was at its highest as well. He was unable to remain seated and asked if he could leave as soon as he sat down. He remained long enough for a very short **Fearlessness** session in order for me to search for the cause of his fear that lead to such an extreme high level of blood pressure, blood counts and anxiety. As it turned out, he was aware of the TMJ dislocation problem but was unable to afford the copayment for the surgery. In addition to his financial worry, he was very self-conscious. He thought that people were always staring at his mouth as it was always open due to the dislocation of his jaw joint. This was not as noticeable as he thought. He was living with a **fearful unknown future**, fearing the way others would judge him if he remained this way for the rest of his life.

Before he left, I arranged for the ENT doctor to see if he could offer Mr. Dodge Don something for his sinusitis. When he saw the ENT doctor, the doctor informed him the dislocated jaw joint could only be fixed by the Maxillofacial Surgeon. However, the ENT doctor offered surgery to assist with his breathing. The very next visit to the clinic, he was very patient and sat calmly. His blood counts were completely normal for the first time. Wow! I was stunned, but remained collected, and turned to his wife and asked, what happened since that last visit? They were so excited because they received a pre-op letter from the ENT doctor. Finally, they thought, the ENT doctor was going to fix his dislocated jaw.

A closer look at the ENT letter showed the pre-op appointment was for sinuses surgery rather than for TMJ (for his jaw), but I could not bear to disappoint him. After a long **Fearlessness** discussion, he accepted and agreed that the sinus surgery could help him with his breathing without having to open his mouth. After the sinus surgery, he became much calmer and more relaxed.

His blood pressure as well as his blood work was better controlled. His leukocytosis level also trended down. Due to the improvement, he is on observation instead of being given further work up or intervention.

Discussion 4:
What was so unusual about Mr. Dodge Don and what was observed? Beside his complaints of bone pain, general weakness and muscle ache, the unusual complaint was that he had trouble breathing as well as the need to open his mouth to breathe. Why was he breathing this way? He was breathing similarly to many **anxiety** patients. The opening of his mouth was partially due to jaw joint issue, but mostly due to his anxiety, his breathing became worse. Due to financial constraint, he was unable to have his jaw joint issue fixed previously. What was he anxious about? The thought that people were always staring at his mouth because it remained opened. He anxiously wanted to have it fixed as he feared to be judged. As he feared to be judged (stared at) his breathing became more difficult and his mouth opened frequently to breathe. Due to the fear of being judged, his anxiety became more frequent and his breathing became difficult causing him to become unable to sit for more than three minutes. The opening of his mouth was barely noticeable when he was calm.   How was his fear resolved? He accepted that the sinus surgery could in fact help with his breathing and in turn help lessen the opening of his mouth.

Words to live by

Taoism:
"To see things in the seed, that is genius."

Chapter 5
Avoidance

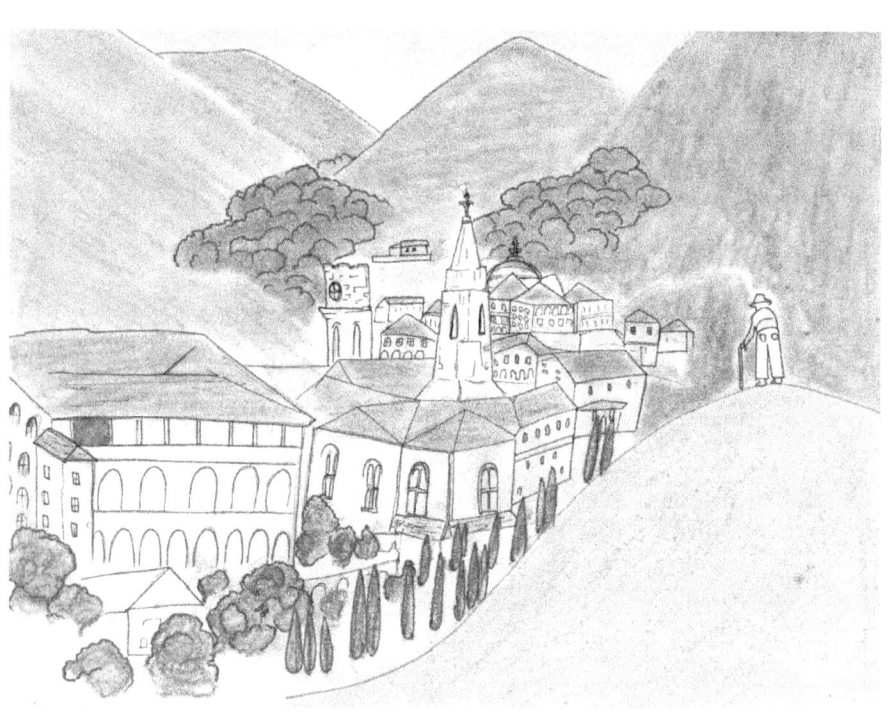

Mr. Kobe Kentucky is a patient who arrived with a long history of back pain. The back pain gradually became worse, so severe that he went to the emergency department. He lost twenty three pounds within the past two months. During the ER visit, the CT scan showed advanced multiple myeloma with possible spinal cord compression. Multiple myeloma is a plasma cell cancer that grows in the bone

When he first came in to evaluate his multiple myeloma, he was **erratic**, **impatient** and **furious** with his primary doctor. He complained that he had gone there about a dozen times and each time his doctor did nothing, but gave him pain medication. He threatened to file a law suit. I managed to calm him down and introduced the concept of **Fearlessness** to reduce his anger.

I asked if he would like to feel better; he replied yes. I explained that he was right to get angry with his primary doctor, but that his health and time were more important than what had happened. As difficult as it was for him, he agreed to let the past go and focus on the present. I reviewed the CT scans with him and confirmed that the cancer had attached to his spinal cord and that there was a chance that he could become paralyse. He was hospitalized right away to expedite the work up and the treatment to prevent his compression from causing further damage.

Tremendous effort was required to persuade him

to be hospitalized. After only one day in the hospital, he requested the doctors to release him because he needed to go home to situate his pets and to pay his bills. He was living with the **fearful unknown future**.

When I met with him in the hospital ward and persuaded him to remain in the hospital, he called a friend to feed his pets. Due to the severity of the disease (his diagnosis was found at the later stage), he began chemotherapy quickly followed by radiation. He returned to the clinic after completing radiation for a follow up. He was grateful that he was able to walk normally without the back pain.

Although his disease was found at an advanced stage, he had a great response to chemotherapy and radiation treatment. Due to the advanced stage of disease however, he was required to continue with oral chemotherapy. He had a difficult time with the oral chemotherapy. He only took the treatment for two days and stopped on his own. As he explained, he started to feel all of the side effects of the medication on the second day. He went through the list of side effects several times and he had each one of them. No doubt, he remained very fearful.

After several more attempts to reduce his **fear**, he eventually agreed to resume treatment. He continued on the same oral chemotherapy treatment without any side effects. Soon after, he was not only able to relinquish his **fear**, but he also made changes in his life. After residing in his house for over thirty years, he made a big decision and moved to a place closer to the hospital. He later shared that his expectation of the future and his outlook on life was filled with more control and was better than ever. He made the best use of his time and was able to enjoy his time to the utmost.   This allowed him to travel, and visit Italy for three weeks on his own and then another three weeks to South America. He continues to do well with plans to travel and revisit Italy.

Discussion 5:
What was learned about Mr. Kobe Kentucky? He was aware that he could become paralyse if he did not start treatment after learning of his diagnosis. Masking his fear, he requested to leave the hospital to care for his pets and to pay his bills. But after completing his introduction treatment, he was able to walk and no longer had back pain.   He began to detach his **fear**. However, he was unable to avoid his fear of the unknown future. He had a difficult time starting his oral chemotherapy. He was unable to tolerate the medication because he experienced all of the side effects of the medication on the second day. No doubt, he remained very **fearful**. How did he overcome his fear? Slowly, he retried the same oral chemotherapy treatment as he recalled how the introduction treatment had helped him. During his second try of the oral chemotherapy medication, he tolerated it without any side

effects. As he gained more control of his **fear**, he also made changes and adjustments in his life. He became more flexible and moved to a place closer to the hospital. His expectation of the future and outlook changed. His life was more fulfilled. He made the best use of his time and was able to enjoy his time to the utmost. He travelled and visited Italy on his own. He continued to make plans to enjoy his life with future travels.

Words to live by

Taoism:
"When I let go of what I am, I become what I might be."

Group II
FEARFUL PAST

Chapter 6
Insomnia

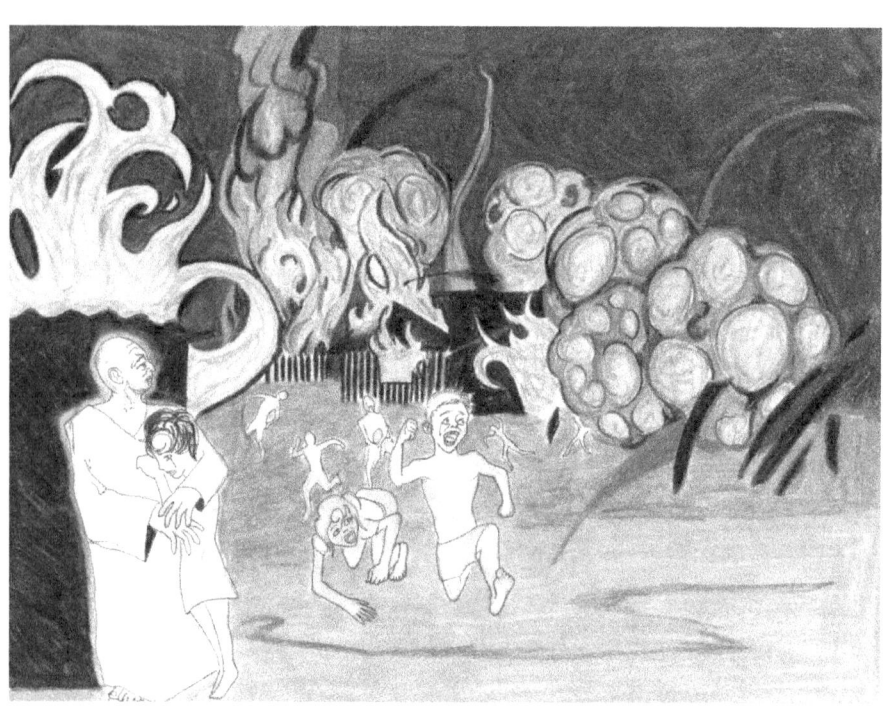

Mr. Pedro Pennsylvania is an elderly patient who has high blood pressure, diabetes, chronic neck pain, rosacea and low blood counts. Only in the last five years had his blood work became abnormal. After obtaining his bone marrow biopsy, he learned that he also has MDS.

His wife usually accompanied him to his doctor appointments. Every time he came in, he complained of **fatigue** and blamed old age. His **fatigue** became worse each visit.

He was introduced to the **Fearlessness** concept to help resolve his fatigue. During the session, his wife disclosed that he had nightmares every night for years. Sometimes his nightmares were worse than others. Within the last year, his nightmares were becoming more real, more frequent, and violent. His wife said she became a "punching bag". She recalled that a couple months ago, he was yelling and fought so violently, that he swung and broke her nose. During the nightmares, he would speak in another language, screaming and apparently fighting hard. After listening to his wife, he started to cry and explained that while he was serving in Vietnam there was a particular incident that haunted him. Even his wife of fifty years was unaware of this incident.

He began his explanation by recalling the incident that happened while he was serving in the Vietnam War. The tragic incident took place when he was ordered to fire directly into a village. When the firing ceased, he entered the village, and realized the people that were killed in the village were mostly kids and the elderly. He was unable to stop sobbing as he related the incident.

At the end of this **Fearlessness** session, he agreed that it was not his fault and what had happened to those village people was in the past. He also accepted that the Vietnamese people, who died during the war, would have forgiven him if they could have met him now because they would see his sorrow and pain. He simply obeyed an order which was his duty. It could have easily been the other way around. He even went as far as asking for their forgiveness during the session. Asking for their forgiveness, he accepted and understood that the incident was in the past. He let go of his guilt.

At the next visit, his blood work, for the first time, was in normal range. Most surprisingly on this visit, Mr. Pedro was not complaining about **fatigue** for the very first time! His wife added that his overall outlook on life since that last visit also changed for the better.

Since his introduction to the **Fearlessness**, he was able to accept his **fearful past** and make peace with himself. He stopped having nightmares and became energized and happy. He continued to do well for two years, then his blood counts trended below normal.

We quickly revisited **Fearlessness** to further

investigate the cause for the downward trend of his blood tests. During this session, he stated that he was very sad and felt that his youngest daughter no longer loved him. This was surprising even to his wife. She was unaware that he felt this way. He felt that his youngest daughter moved away to another state to be as far away as possible from he and his wife. They tried to contact her, but she refused to release her phone numbers to them. They had not spoken for over two years. He could not understand why his daughter would choose her husband, whom he thought was not good for her, over them. He was living with the **fearful past** that his daughter made the decision to lose contact with them based on what happened in the past.

After our session, he accepted that it was important to give her time and space. As soon as he accepted this, he was able to have peace and his blood counts started to improve. His blood work remained stable without dropping below normal range. On the following visit, his blood work reached its highest point of normal range. Both Mr. Pedro and his wife were extremely happy on this particular visit. After learning the result, he informed me that over the weekend his youngest daughter finally called and spoke to him for a very long time. She agreed to remain in touch. Since then, his blood work continued to remain in the normal range. Time between his visits was extended and he was able to remain on extended follow ups without further treatment to date.

Discussion 6:

What was the significance about Mr. Pedro Pennsylvania? For years, Mr. Pennsylvania had been having nightmares. His nightmares became worse and became more real. Mr. Pedro blamed himself for firing and killing the village people who were mostly the elderly and children.   Feeling guilt for wrongfully killing the Vietnamese, he was unable to rest well at nights; this was the source of his fatigue. Accepting this was all in the past, he asked forgiveness. He let go of his **fear** and guilt. He stopped having nightmares and became energized and happy. Letting go of fear took some time, the loss of contact with his youngest daughter restarted his fear and guilt. He felt unloved by his youngest daughter who moved away to another state.   Because he once thought that his son in law was not good for his daughter, Mr. Pennsylvania felt guilt and blamed himself for her reason for moving so far away. Once he understood, he was able to let go of his fear and guilt. He accepted that he had to give his youngest daughter time and space. In the end, he was happy and regained control of his life.

Words to live by

Taoism:
"To the mind that is still, the whole universe surrenders."

Chapter 7
Pain

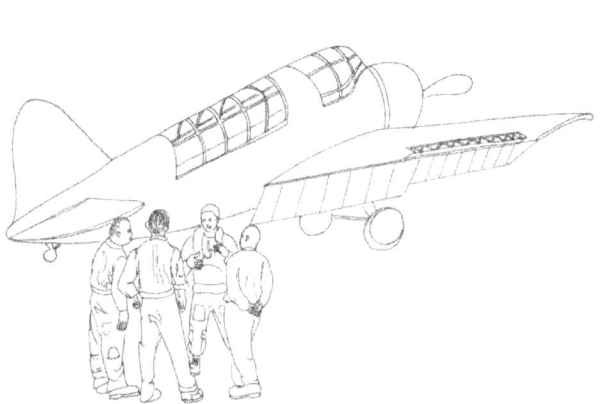

Mr. Rhode Island is an elderly patient. He did not have a very long list of diseases, but was diagnosed with prostate cancer over ten years ago. He received radiation without chemotherapy for his prostate cancer.   Hormonal therapy was started just three years ago. The prostate cancer responded well to the treatment.   Mr. Rhode however, had daily headaches for over sixty five years since serving in WW II. He was seen to evaluate for depressed blood cell lines and especially for progressively worsened fatigue and headaches. His blood cell counts much like pancytopenia had been depressed for over five years without much change.

On his first visit, he presented himself as an extraordinary pleasant patient. He came in with his wife who was very caring and understood and knew him well. Both were well groomed and he was especially crisp and sharply dressed. During his assessment, he asked why he was always fatigued, weak, and lacking energy. He denied any known infections. He was offered **Fearlessness** to search for the causes of his fatigue, weakness, and lack of energy.

During the **Fearlessness-**session, I learned that he was a very successful and held many high positions during his working years, but was always fatigued and had frequent headaches. His wife revealed that he loved working, but seldom enjoyed anything else.

As the searching sessions continued, he unfolded

an underlying guilt that he carried with him over sixty five years from the time he was a pilot instructor during WW II. He choked up with tears of guilt, as well as anger as he recalled the loss of sixteen pilots. He was angry because he thought the pilots were not serious when he was teaching them with clear and important instruction. He continued to choke up and expressed anger as he recalled this time. He had purposely failed pilots but he was forced to re-instruct them because they needed pilots for the war effort. He went as far as having pilots explicitly repeated his instructions, like a recital. Even with the new instruction, he felt that some of them should not have been passed to fly. He vividly recalled going up in a flight of nine planes; his plane was the only one that made it back. This occurred in the thick clouds of Alaska. The pilots disregarded his warnings and lost their lives. He claimed to have suffered a minor head injury in this experience. The loss of his fellow pilots, although an accident, was something that haunted him for over sixty five years. This guilt and anger were with him since WW II and was the source of his headaches and fatigue. He had continued to live in this haunted **past.**

When we concluded our session, Mr. Rhode Island turned to me tearfully and said in his gentle voice that he had attended many psychological therapies over forty years, but was unable to release his frustration, anger and guilt until now. He graciously thanked me which made an incredible imprint on my life. When we ended our first and only session, Mr. Rhode Island was referred for bone marrow biopsy. He was unable to keep the appointment. He was hospitalized for a heart attack and passed away one week prior to his appointment.

Discussion 7:

Why did Mr. Rhode Island had headaches that occurred daily for over 65 years? He had an underlying guilt that he carried within him from the time he was a pilot instructor during **WW II**. He felt responsible for his pilot students' deaths. Why was his responsibility filled with so much guilt and anger?   He felt angry because the pilots were not serious when he was trying to teach them, and he thought this was the reason that had caused their deaths. He had failed pilots, but he was forced to re-instruct them because they needed pilots for the war effort. He even changed his teaching method and went as far as having the pilots explicitly repeat the instructions. Even with this new method, he felt that some of them should not have been passed to fly. Was Mr. Rhode able to resolve his fear? Finally, near the end of his life, Mr. Rhode became aware of his fear (responsible for the loss of his pilots) and was able to resolve this fear. He then expressed the release of this frustration. It is expected that his headaches would have lessened, but his sudden passing was unable to confirm.

Words to live by

John 14:27:
Peace I leave with you, my peace I give unto you: not as the world giveth, give I unto you. Let not your heart be troubled, neither let it be afraid.

Group III

FEARFUL PAST and UNKNOWN FUTURE

Chapter 8
Fatigue

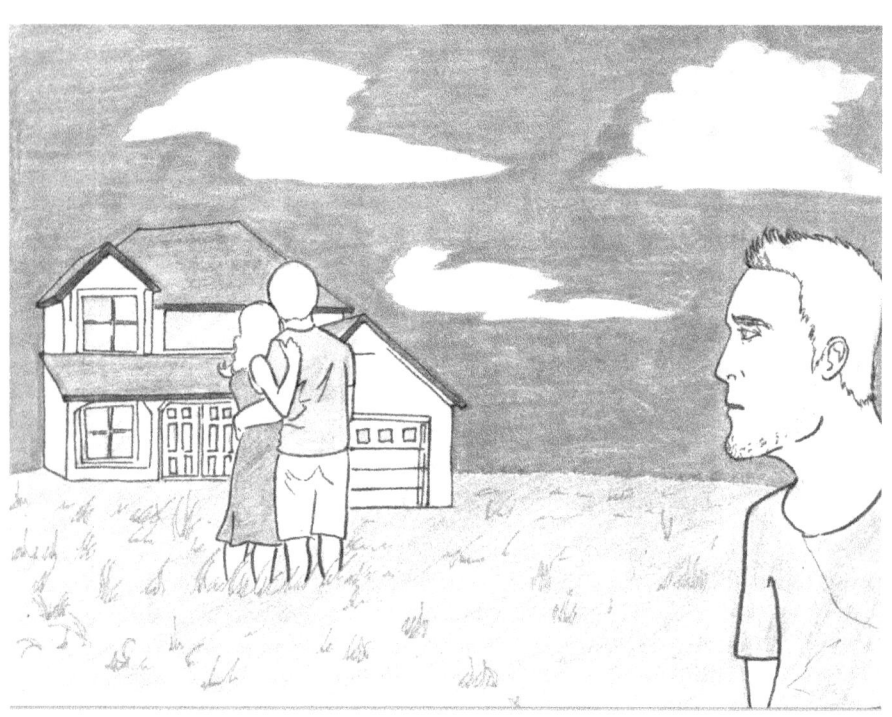

Mr. Dale Dakota is a patient who suffers from worsening fatigue and restlessness of unknown cause. This was thought to be related to his low blood counts from his primary doctor. After reviewing his blood work, he was referred for a bone marrow biopsy. The result of the bone marrow biopsy revealed that he had myelodysplasic syndrome (MDS).

Each and every time Mr. Dakota came in, he complained of fatigue and the inability to sleep at night. Each visit, his fatigue and restlessness were more intense. To search for the cause and to reduce his fatigue and restlessness, the concept of **Fearlessness** was introduced. What was uncovered through **Fearlessness** was very interesting. He had been afraid of losing his wife, not to an illness, but to another man. Mr. Dakota had several divorces in the past. For the past two years, he had done everything in his power to save his marriage. He was financially successful. He had nice cars and a beautiful home. As a last resort to save his marriage, he had taken his wife on a fourteen day first class, Hawaiian cruise. As soon as they returned, she filed for divorce. She handed him the paper work on Valentine's Day.

Each time he returned for his follow up, his fatigue and restlessness remained unimproved. He often didn't want to do his blood work either. This condition remained unchanged until I tried my "Lyanne's car" analogy. I began by asking him to pick out his dream car. He picked a

Ferrari. I then asked him to pretend that he could transform himself into this car. This Ferrari would take him anywhere he needed to go. Then one day, he had to be at a place he really wanted to go. On his way there, he was told that the road had been blocked and it would be impossible to get through. It was not certain when the road would re-open. What would he do then? His answer was to try and find another way to get there. This answer was a very common one among my past "worrier-warrior" type patients. Really, there was no right, nor wrong answer.

I explained to Mr. Dakota that by driving around to find a new route, he could have gotten lost. He would need lots of time and gasoline because he would eventually run out if he continued to drive aimlessly to find his way. Even if gasoline was available, he was not going to get there because it was impossible to do so. The bottom line, it was **impossible to get there.**

This scenario was much like his life. He spent lots of time and energy over and over again, like the Ferrari circling around and around the impossible. His wife had made up her mind to leave. The road was blocked until she decided she wanted him back. The impossible road would remain impossible. He was burning his energy like fuel and therefore he constantly felt fatigued and unhappy.

On the next visit, he came in with a smile and stated that he had changed. He no longer wanted to strangle the man, once a friend that stole his wife. He made peace with himself. I was stunned and excited to hear this, and saw him smile for the first time. Finally, I thought, he got it! When I glanced at his blood work, only a portion of the blood work had improved. I later understood why.

As we continued with our discussion, he mentioned that he had done something very nice for his ex-wife, and that she had no idea. He was the main donor to the church collection to help his ex-wife with the burial of her grandchildren. He was upset with his ex-wife for not mentioning him at all as the step-grandfather in the obituary. The following visit, he related that he had paid for a car rental so that his ex-wife's daughter could attend the burial of her father (who also had recently passed away).   He was upset because he wanted to attend the burial, but was not invited. He was unable to overcome his fear and continued to hold on to the impossible **past**, living in the impossible future with his ex-wife.

Discussion 8:
Why did Mr. Dakota complain of fatigue and the inability to sleep? He was afraid of losing his wife for two years and at the same time was in denial.
   From the "Lyanne's car" analogy, he uncovered that he was driving aimlessly, like the Ferrari circling around and around the impossible. The road was blocked until his ex-wife would decide she wanted him back. The road remained blocked. As he continued to choose to be in

denial, he did things hoping his ex-wife would accept him back. Became the main donor to the church collection to help his ex-wife with the burial of her grandchildren, he expected to be mentioned as the step-grandfather in the obituary from his ex-wife. Then, he paid for a car rental so that his ex-wife's daughter could attend the burial of her father.   He was upset because he was not invited to the burial.   In the end, he was unable to overcome his **fear** and continued to hold on to the **past, living in the impossible future** with his ex-wife.

Words to live by

Voltaire (Writer, philosopher, 1694-1778): The man who leaves money to charity in his will is only giving away what no longer belongs to him.

Chapter 9
Nyctophobia

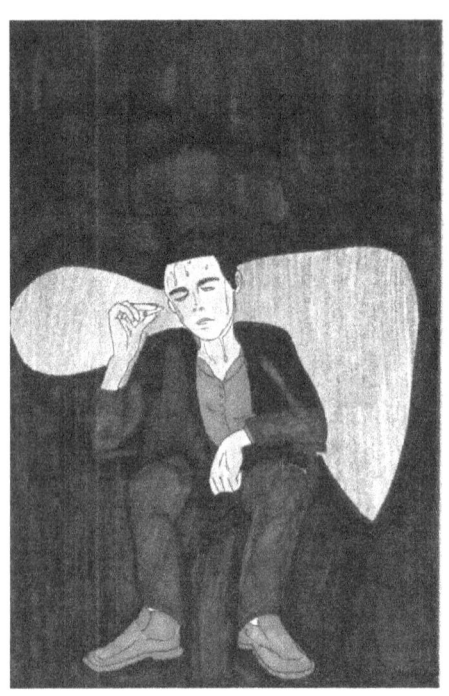

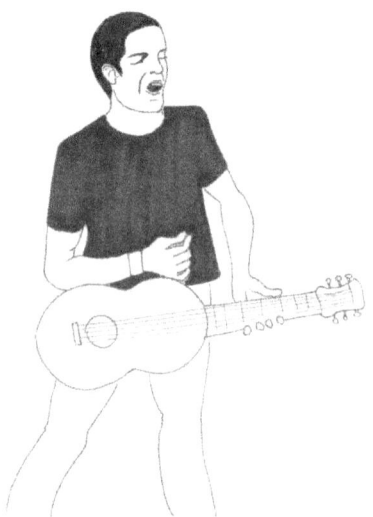

Mr. Romy Zero is a patient who had a long list of diseases including a liver problem, hepatitis C. He was seen to evaluate his high level of iron further evaluated. On his first visit, he presented as a very well groomed individual wearing a stylish hat. His wife who accompanied him was much the opposite due to her casual appearance. He was **impatient** and wanted to quickly leave stating that he felt fine and did not need to be seen. His wife was anxious and appeared to be uptight about something. They bickered frequently during this first visit.

After reviewing his blood work, he was sent to have additional blood work. The blood work result confirmed that he had hemachromatosis. Hemachromatosis is a disorder of too much iron accumulation in the body which can lead to organ toxicity.

Mr. Zero and his wife continued to bicker on the following visit. They were offered **Fearlessness** to reduce his impatience and her agitation. During the **Fearlessness** session, his wife complained that he smoked too much. He smoked at least two packs a day while she only smoked one pack a day. They were spending too much money on cigarettes and she was hoping he would slow down since they were on a tight budget. She added that he spent all of his time, day and night in his room, coming out only to eat. His explanation was that he could not sleep through the night. He awoke at one AM and couldn't get back to sleep.

Not until the second **Fearlessness** session, he began to reveal his tragic and horrific past. While he was serving in Vietnam, his wife had a baby. The baby required surgery so he was sent back to the states. The baby not only required one surgery, but two. The baby did not survive the second surgery. He decided to return to Vietnam to continue his tour and volunteered as a mine detector. He performed mine sweeping early every morning. One day a small bus exploded after he cleared the road. He was not at that scene, but his friend described everything in detail to him. His friend vividly described the pregnant woman and her fetus. His friend found the fetus and buried both of them. Shortly after that incident, Mr. Zero encountered a Vietnamese street vendor. The vendor asked if he would like to purchase a dead baby monkey which was skewed to a long stick. As he described, the baby monkey reminded him of a human baby because it was also small and white due to the removal of the skin.

As our discussion continued, he unveiled another frightening event in his past which resulted in his **fear** of darkness.   As part of a minesweeper crew, Mr. Zero served as a tank guard. He had to stay up at night making sure the enemy would not sneak up on them. As he patrolled, he constantly checked his gun to be sure it was loaded and that extra ammunition remained handy. This resulted in a nonstop nervousness, and a fear that his weapon would somehow vanish. He also constantly feared the presence of the enemy to the point that he urinated in his pants just from the sound of the wind.   At dawn, his **fear** disappeared and his rapid heartbeat would slow allowing him to feel relaxed, his unstoppable sweating also diminished. This **fear** would return with the first sign of night. This continued after the war as he continued to live in the **past** this **fear** had kept him awake at night for years. He had seen many psychotherapists, taken courses in psychology, but was unable to release this **fear**.

As tragic and horrific as was his past, he recognized that the events were in the past and he managed to make changes. He started to play his guitar again which he had not done for over thirty five years. He also became more loving. His wife however was unable to accept his sudden changes. As she explained, he was cold for over thirty five years and suddenly he opened doors for her, sang and helped around the house. She cried and asked if he could return to his old self. She was very **fearful** of living in a **unknown future** and suspected that his illness had gotten worse instead of accepting that he finally had let go of his past. He remained functional and started to care for himself by eating healthy. He continues to be stable at the present time.

Discussion 9:
What was learned about Mr. Romy Zero? He was impatient, up tight and remained awake at night for years. He nervously correlated his **fear** of

darkness to his **fear** for his life. With the first sign of night, the **fear** and frightening emotions returned from the time he served as a tank guard. As he patrolled, he constantly repeated checking his gun fearing that his weapon would somehow vanish. He was constantly feeling someone was there. This **fear** escalated to the point that he urinated in his pants repeatedly just from the sound of the wind. Was he able to resolve his fear? As he realized and accepted these horrific events were in the past, he was able to resolve his fear. He became more loving as he overcame his **fear**. His wife however remained fearful and was unable to accept his sudden changes. As she explained, he was cold for over thirty five years and suddenly he opened doors for her, sang and helped around the house. She cried and asked if he could return to his old self. She was very **fearful** of living in an **unknown future** and suspected his illness had gotten worse instead of accepting that he finally let go of his past.

Words to live by

Proverbs 17:22:
A merry heart doeth good like a medicine: but a broken spirit drieth the bones.

Chapter 10
Angry

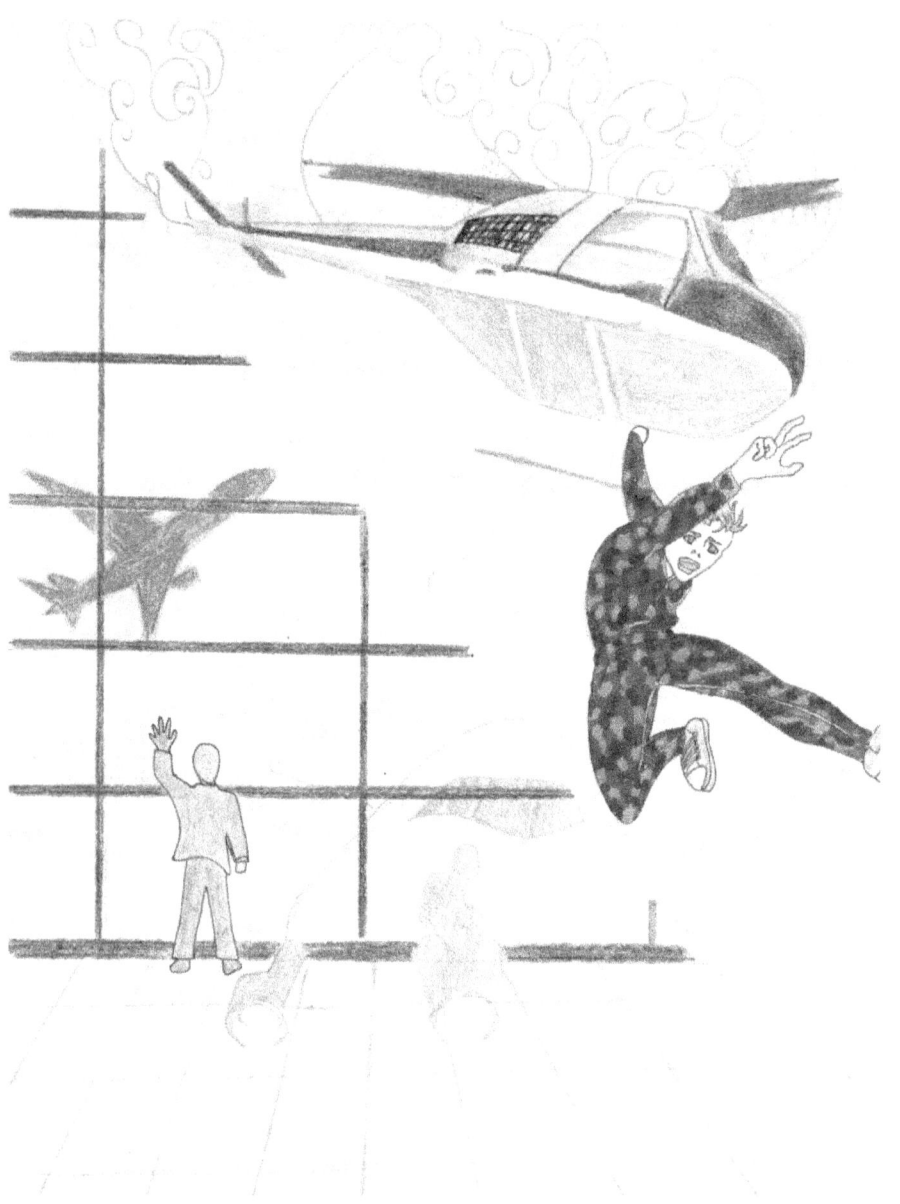

Mr. Kirk Kansas is a patient, who like many patients, had a long list of medical diseases. He was referred to be evaluated for erythrocytosis. He appeared to be very quiet on his first visit. He wore a long beard and was very thin. After reviewing his blood work, he was referred to have an additional work up. The additional tests indicated that he had a disease known as Gaisbock's disease, hypovolemia or tress erythrocytosis. There are no known treatment guidelines for Gaisbock's syndrome, other than to drink more water to expand the vascular volume.

During follow up, he did not have any physical complaints, but complained about his next door neighbors. He would express his animosity toward his neighbors. He thought that they were constantly watching his house. He also expressed his distrust of them since he had seen them using sewage water to water their plants and then sell them as organic fruits and vegetables. He suspected that they also served these vegetables in their local family dinners. He was offered **Fearlessness** to search for the cause of his fear when he came in for a follow up and appeared angry and spacy, not in his usual self.

As the session proceeded, he unveiled his horrific and guilt filled past. While serving in Vietnam, a chain of misfortunes repeatedly happened to him. He recalled his first incident as he was asleep when all of a sudden he had gotten blown out of his bunker. Soon after that incident, his parachute jump plane was "hit" as he was making his jump. His legs were tangled swinging back and forth from the burning plane and he thought at the time that his life was about to end. Shortly thereafter, he was thrown out of a truck while he was delivering ammunition. It was blown up! Yet, those incidents were nothing compared to what he witnessed as ARVNS (Army of the Republic of Vietnam) tortured "CHARLIE" (Vietcong). The ARVNS tortured "CHARLIE" by shooting off one finger at a time during integration. The same ARVNS continued by cutting off "Charlie's" private part and stuffing it in his mouth. They then left him on the road. He asked angrily, "Why did the ARVNs perform such torture on their own people!" For years, he was unable to be in a large crowd or around unfamiliar people especially Asian; particularly the Vietnamese. He was living in a **fearful unknown future**. He expressed that if he was in line and there was another person behind him, he would immediately step out of line because he did not trust what that person would do next. I found out that his neighbor, whom he constantly complained about, was also Asian. His distrust and anger at those horrific events of his past continued to live within him. He continued living in the **fearful past!**

As the **Fearlessness** session continued, his fearful past started to unfold with guilt. His misfortune turned into good fortune when he over slept and missed his flight home in the Fall of 1978. He recalled vividly his bunk mate waking him stating that his plane was leaving. He hurriedly ran after the plane as it was taking off.

He felt angrily at himself for oversleeping and missing a chance of going home. The very next day he learned that the plane had crashed. His distrust, anger and fear were so deeply ingrained that his daily life from that point was lived with constant reminders of the past. After several more months of **Fearlessness**, he began to slowly recognize and accept that the events were in the past and slowly began to show improvement. He shaved off his beard, quit smoking and started to gain a bit more weight.

After changing his diet to a healthier one, he joined the VFW (*Veterans of Foreign Wars*). His blood work also started to show improvement. He continued to this day to make little changes with each session and to show improvement. He participates in welcoming service men and women back home. He thought that was the least he could do since men of the Vietnam Era received no such welcome.

Discussion 10:
What was revealed about Mr. Kirk Kansas? He had trust and anger issues. His anger and distrust became part of his life. He was unable to be in large crowd or around unfamiliar people. Why was he so distrustful and angry? His distrust and anger were the result of his experiences that he encountered during the horrific events while he was fighting during the Vietnam War. He witnessed as ARVNS (Army of the Republic of Vietnam) tortured "CHARLIE" (Vietcong) by shooting off one finger at a time during

integration and cutting off "Charlie's" private part and stuffing it in his mouth. He did not understand why the ARVNs performed such torture on their own people! He continued living in the **fearful past** with his distrust. He would immediately step out of line if another person was behind him when he was in line. He do not trust what that person would do next. How did he overcome his fear? Very slowly, he recognized and accepted that the events were in the past, he began to make changes. He shaved off his beard, started to eat healthy and joined the VFW.

Words to live by

Matthew 5:44:
But I say unto you, Love your enemies, bless them that curse you, do good to them that hate you, and pray for them which despitefully use you, and persecute you.

Chapter 11
Hate

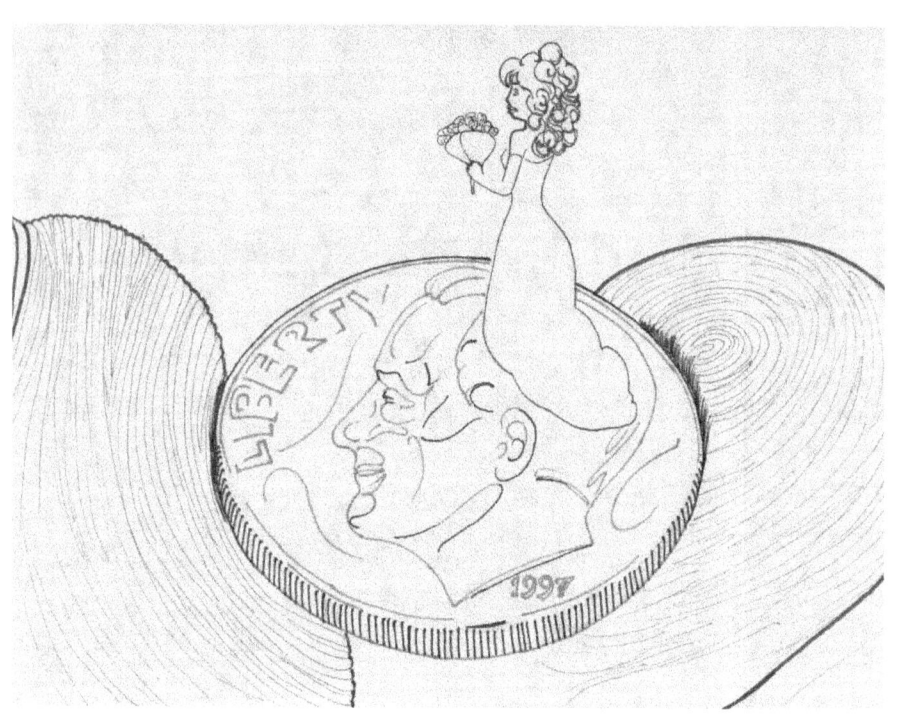

Ms. Donna Lisa is a patient with an extremely long list of medical problems along with twenty past surgeries. Besides her existing problems, she was referred to be evaluated for chronic neutropenia. Neutropenia is an abnormally low number of white blood cells, cells that help the body fight infection. Her neutropenia was first discovered in the 1980's, but she failed follow ups until she moved to California. She had been receiving treatment with Neupogen for several months. Her blood counts had not responded to any treatment. Her doctor, without any other options, switched her to the newest treatment. Again, her treatment was failing. She showed no improvement. She required more frequent treatment, moving from once a month to twice a month. Due to her failing response, she sought a second opinion at our clinic.

On her first visit, she was very **anxious**, **depressed** and **emotional**. She was offered **Fearlessness** to search for her fear and to reduce her anxiety. I recalled this first visit because she was very emotional. She was unable to express herself without getting tearful and angry. As the session proceeded, she unveiled that she hated men because they cheat and lie. In her past, she married and divorced seven times. She married "at the drop of a dime". Her first marriage was at age nineteen. She got married simply to be able to move out of state. After having a son and daughter, she got divorced. She then joined the army and married a civilian (who she claimed raped her). During this time, she had sought help on this rape case, but the army court found her at fault. She felt betrayed by the military. She felt the military took the civilian's side instead of hers. She then divorced and married for the third time. The third marriage also did not last long. She then married a man who was twenty years younger than her. Of all her marriages, she loved this man the most, but his parents and family were difficult to deal with; hence she divorced for the fourth time. She married a fifth time at age forty four. This marriage, she claimed was the worst. She again claimed she was raped and abused. Soon after she got her fifth divorce, she married a minister. This sixth marriage did not last long either. She divorced the minister who she claimed cheated on her. She then married and divorced for the seventh time. She claimed that this seventh husband also raped her.

As our session continued, the tragedy began to unfold. As it turned out, her childhood experiences were tragic. She was molested at age five by her uncle who baby sat. The man whom she was told was her dad, turned out to be another stepfather. She did not find out until visiting him at age thirteen; he also tried to molest her. She later found that her mother had hidden the truth because she did not want to be tied down to a service man, fearing that she would be left a widow. Her three siblings were all from different fathers, for her mother had several marriages herself. Not only was her past a tragic one, her present situation was as tragic as her past. Her daughter was molested by her cousin at age twelve.

Her son who was only in his twenties, never got married, but had at least twelve known children, all were from different women. Out of twelve grandchildren, two granddaughters were abandoned by their mother at birth. They were raised by her since her son was in and out of jail for selling and doing drugs. She had to constantly bail her son out from jail. She was also running into financial problems because of her girls' troubles. They were not returning home at night, partying and crashing her cars.   She continued seeing her old oncologist while she was coming to see me.

To my surprise, after the first session, she stated that she needed to let go of her son's troubles and the granddaughters' problems. She decided that she would not bail them out since they were already adults. They should learn to resolve their own problems. Since then, her blood counts started to show great improvement. Her blood counts began to stabilize. Her previous treatment schedule (every two weeks) with her old oncologist was extended to every two months. Not only was her old oncologist surprised, but so was her cardiologist, who did not understand why suddenly her blood pressure was under control. Previously, she was unable to be in elevators with others. She would avoid movie theatres and crowded places, even the grocery store.   She only shopped late at night or early morning, no more than twenty minutes at a time. She was living with a **fearful past and fearful unknown future.**

Besides worrying about her son and her two granddaughters, she had to deal with her high and low moments. She would go on a shopping spree on her high moment and the very next day return the items. As dramatic and complicated as she was, she was a quick learner and understood that she was able to control her high and low spending moods. She was able to save enough money to travel to Hawaii and stay three weeks to see her family and friends. She started focusing on her life, letting go of the problems of her grown son and the two granddaughters. She continued to improve. Her interval of treatment was extended allowing her to continue to make plans to travel to different parts of the country and world to visit her friends.

Discussion 11:
What was Ms. Donna Lisa issues? She was constantly searching for love and belonging. Irrationally, she married seven times. She married men "at the drop of a dime".   As she searched for love, she claimed she was raped by several of her ex-husbands. She hated men because they cheat and lie. Unfortunately, her past and present were very troubled and tragic. She was surrounded by the fear of the past and fear of the unknown future. She worried

constantly about her son who was in his twenties, constantly in and out of jail for selling and doing drugs; never got married, and had at least twelve known children, all from different women. She constantly encountered the troubles caused by the two granddaughters. Not only was her past very tragic, she was constantly afraid of what would happen to her next. She was unable to be in elevators with others. She would avoid movie theatres and crowded places, even the grocery store.   She only shopped late at night or early morning, no more than twenty minutes at a time. She was constantly in fear.   As tragic, dramatic and complicated as she was, she learned to overcome her **fear** to gain freedom from her disease and fulfil her life. She accepted that she needed to focus on herself instead of her son and her granddaughters. As soon as she began to make adjustments and changes to improve her life style, her treatment also improved. Previously, her spending was uncontrollable. After her adjustment, she was able to save enough money to travel to Hawaii and stay three weeks to see her family and friends. She continued to make plans to travel which was not an easy task for she was once very fearful of crowds.

Words to live by

John 4:18
There is no fear in love; but perfect love casteth out fear: because fear hath torment. He that feareth is not made perfect in love.

Chapter 12
Denial

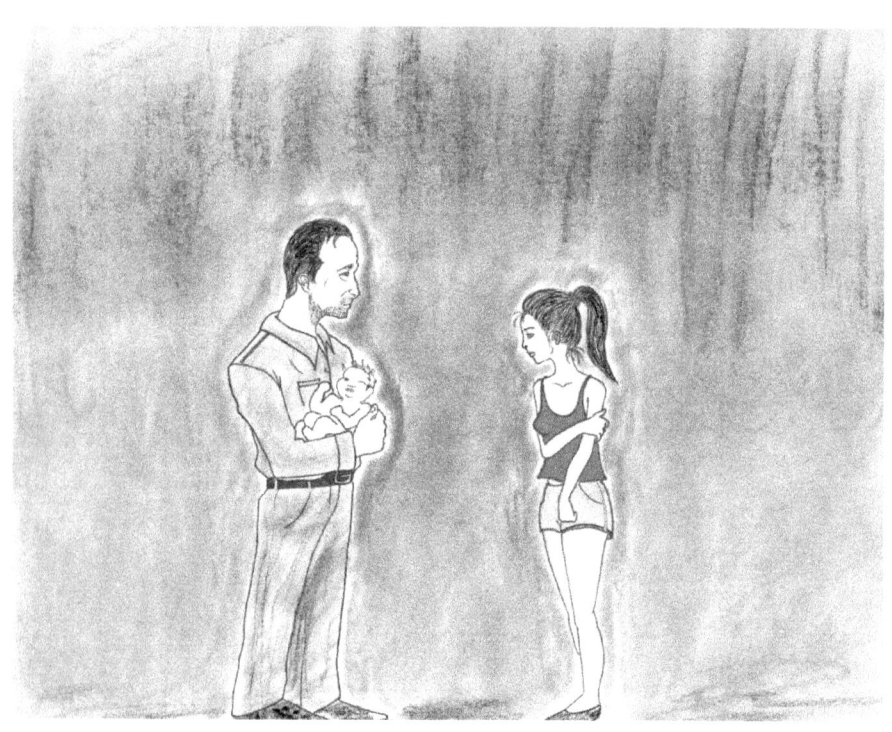

Mr. Kansas Ken is a patient with a long list of medical diseases including Non-Hodgkin Lymphoma. Lymphoma is a cancer type that involves the blood or the immune system. Mr. Kansas previously completed chemotherapy treatment at a different facility and was considered in remission. After moving, he transferred his care to our facility for continued observation. For almost three years, he always had a calm demeanour, was quiet and extremely pleasant, and had no complaints. Just passing his three year mark, he suddenly began to show prominent signs of **worry**, **distress** and **anxiety**. Soon these symptoms became more frequent. To reduce the symptoms, he was introduced to the concept of **Fearlessness**.

During the session, he unveiled a very tragic and painful sadness that had haunted him. For years, he had been smoking marijuana every evening prior to going to bed in order to sleep. Without it, he would remain awake all night thinking about his tragic past and experience stress related to his only child, a daughter, who was a drug addict. As a teenager, she delivered an unhealthy and deformed baby without functional organs. The baby was kept alive by an assisted machine, and only survived a very short period of time. He choked up with tears as he remembered holding the baby. He was heartbroken, wishing he could exchange his life for the baby's. For years, the baby's death haunted him. He recently discovered that his daughter had reunited with this baby's dad who had been released from jail a few months before. He had been afraid of this reunion as well as of his daughter's continued drug abuse. He had not spoken to her much, but suspected that she had been using drugs, since he noticed that she had lots of energy and was up all night and not getting much sleep. He had threatened his daughter by saying if he saw the boyfriend around the house he would shoot him.

When I asked about his wife's concerns, he implied that they were on separate pages. He had a very difficult time understanding his wife and what she was really conveying. She would say "yes" when she really meant "no". His wife and daughter had never gotten along. His wife usually ignored his concerns and went on with her life as if there was no problem.

At this point, I realized that he was carrying this tremendous burden alone, and his wife was very much in denial. He had a very difficult time accepting and relinquishing the past. He continued to live in the horrific past! Within three weeks, he returned with a painful swollen leg. I noticed his high levels of stress and worry about his daughter. A lump was observed which progressed into a recurrence of lymphoma. I expedited the work and offered treatment. Against my advice, his wife offered to seek an alternative treatment with herbal medicine. He agreed because he longed for her acknowledgment and support. He was unaware that she was still very much in denial of his cancer recurrence. Was he ready to accept the recurrence?   He agreed to remain under my supervision with follow ups every month. During this time we continued with the **Fearlessness** session. At each follow up, I waited for him to resume treatment.

He remained reluctant to resume chemotherapy for the next three months. He could not convince his wife that the herbal treatment from Japan was not working. The lump continued to grow causing tremendous swelling and producing excruciating pain. He explained that his wife forcefully insisted he continued with the herbal tea, for it needed more time. As the pain was getting worse and the swelling horrendously larger, he realized he needed to focus on himself, not his wife's wishes. He also recognized that his daughter's situation was in the past. He quickly focused on his present problem and accepted that his cancer had returned. As he gained more courage, he was hoping he wouldn't lose his wife's support. He told her he would stop drinking herbal tea and resume chemotherapy.

The lump shrunk down to half the size after only two chemotherapy treatments. He was overly excited and happy. He then began to have second thoughts; maybe the herbal tea had worked, and he did not need to go to chemotherapy. He had very bad experience with his previous chemotherapy treatment. He was very sick through the whole treatment.

To his amazement, his tolerance to chemotherapy

was easier this time. He was slightly fatigued for a day or two.   He hesitantly asked if he was receiving the same chemotherapy.   I assured him that we used the same drugs which resulted in his remission three years ago. He admitted he was psychologically prepared and relaxed during this treatment because he was focused and able to reduce his stress. He was ecstatic at being functional while undergoing his current treatment. He added that he reduced the amount of marijuana he smoked. He became more relaxed because his twenty five year old daughter moved out and had found a job. He still continued to smoke cigarettes, and claimed smoking cigarettes helped him to relax. After receiving chemotherapy over a period of seven months, a PET scan showed great improvement. He requested a break from chemotherapy because he began to have some mild side effects, but agreed to proceed with radiation in order for his leg to maximize treatment.

He returned after the two months break from chemotherapy, and a CT scans showed shrinkage of his leg lesion, but picked up several new small lesions in his lungs. Immediately, I expedited arrangements for a lung biopsy. He refused, stating that these spots in his lung had been there for years. After we rechecked and compared his previous PET/CT, he remained certain and stated that those spots had been there for years. Was he now ready to accept this new finding as well as the recurrence of his lymphoma? Again, he remained reluctant to perform a biopsy. His refusal was undoubtedly **fear** of accepting reality. We proceeded with two months of radiation to obtain maximum shrinkage of his lower leg lesions. Upon completion, after much sessions of **Fearlessness** he agreed to proceed with a lung biopsy.

One week prior to his biopsy appointment, he experienced chest discomfort for which he sought urgent care. He returned to our emergency department and was cleared for a heart problem. He then had CT scans which showed that the lung lesions had grown and had attached themselves to the chest wall. By this time, his anxiety had escalated requiring admission. During the hospital stay, he was worried about everything including what type of chemotherapy he would have and if it would make him sick. After several lengthy discussions, he eventually became calm and was stable enough to have a biopsy at outpatient clinic. When he returned after the biopsy, he revealed that he had been having financial stress and that his daughter was jobless and pregnant again. By this time, his health was in worse shape and the lung lesions were growing. He was too weak; hence he decided to proceed with hospice care and passed away shortly thereafter.

Discussion 12:
How did Mr. Ken Kansas living his life in denial? For years, he had been smoking marijuana every

evening in order to sleep. Without it, he would remain awake all night thinking about his only child, a daughter, who was a drug addict. As a teenager, she delivered an unhealthy and deformed baby without functional organs and the baby only survived a very short period of time. He was heartbroken, wishing he could exchange his life for the baby. For years, the baby's death haunted him. Beside Mr. Kansas' denial, his wife was also in constant denial as well. She was in denial with her daughter's issues and his cancer coming back which caused much delay in his treatment and caused his progression. As the result of not being able to let go of his daughter's issues, Mr. Kansas became depressed as well as **fearful** to accept his reality. He concealed his pain and reality with marijuana and denials. In the end, he remained in denial as long as he could to avoid his **fear** of the dreadful reality.

Words to live by

Taoism:
"To realize that you do not understand is a virtue; not to realize that you do not understand is a defect."

Chapter 13
Sadness

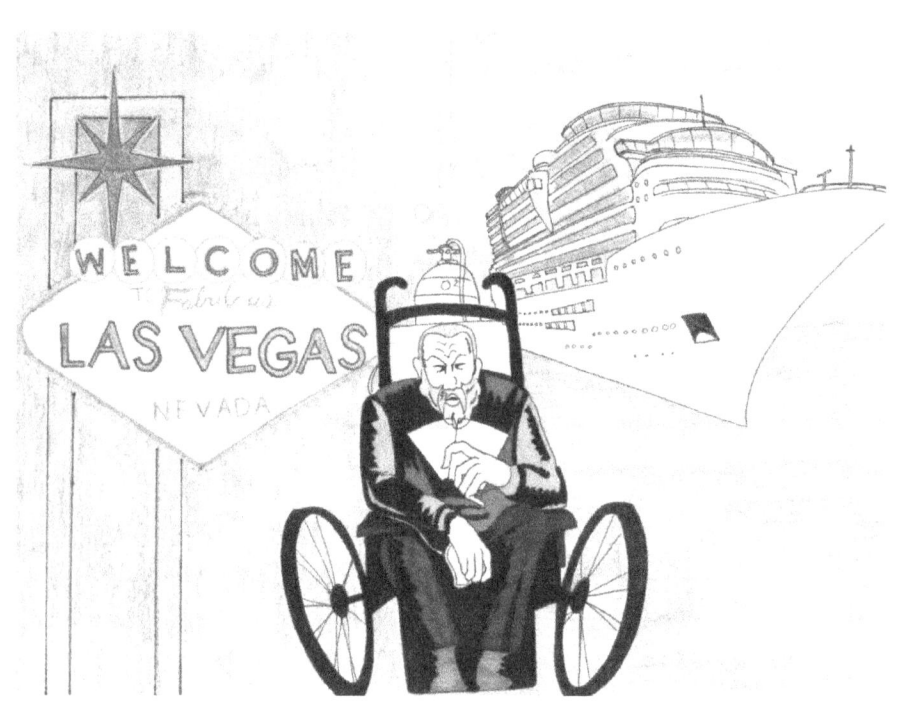

Mr. Diego Delaware is a patient with a long history of heavy smoking. His wife had passed away a year before. While living alone in Northern California, his shortness of breath became worse. It became so severe that he was eventually was unable to breathe and was brought to the emergency room by his neighbor. The ER physician obtained a chest X-ray and found a mass. He also had weight loss of 25 pounds. His daughter who was living in Southern California learned the unfortunate news, and quickly moved him in with her in order to provide care.

When he was first seen, he was very **nervous**, **scared** and was wearing a nasal oxygen cannula while sitting in a wheel chair.   He remained very fearful during this first visit wondering what was going to happen to him.   He recently learned that the mass from the chest X-ray looked like lung cancer. He was quickly sent for additional imaging and later a biopsy to confirm the findings.

Unfortunately, he was found to have late stage (stage IV) lung cancer. Chemotherapy was quickly provided along with the **Fearlessness** to help reduce his anxiety and fear. He remained very anxious and fearful during chemotherapy. He was near a breakdown point having trouble breathing even while on canal oxygen. Recalling this extensive session, I asked him a series of questions. I asked him why he wouldn't let me help him. Was he afraid of dying? To my surprise, he answered that he was not afraid of dying because he wanted to be with his wife. He added that the past two years had been very difficult because his wife was diagnosed with breast cancer and had a terrible time undergoing chemotherapy. She could not tolerate chemotherapy and was only able to complete two cycles. He thought that was why she died a year ago.   His daughter concurred that he often spoke to her as if she was still around in the house. I then asked him if he was having a hard time with the side effects. He replied that he was not, but he just wanted to be able to complete the next cycle of treatments. He recalled that his wife was unable to do that so at that point. I realized then that he was fighting to be able to complete the chemotherapy course.   He was living with a **fearful past and fearful unknown future**!

As the session and discussion continued, he slowly came to understand the need to stay focused and try to take one day at a time. He also understood the need to avoid revisiting his wife's problems which caused pain and sadness. He suddenly broke down crying and said that this particular session was really what he needed.   It was really for him and not the cancer. Since then, he remained emotionally stable. He became very relaxed and strong, despite several hospitalizations, including the placement of a chest tube to help with the drainage of lung fluid. He continued with months of chemotherapy treatments.

His cancer remained stable for over a year. Throughout his treatment, his daughter provided great support. As busy as she was, she would arrange to take him to Las Vegas to see shows, and other events, including a day cruise.   He related later that his time with his daughter provided the most enjoyment he ever had. During the last two months, prior to his passing, he was so calm and collected that he requested to remain at home, on his own, with hospice care.

Discussion 13:
What was Mr. Diego Delaware most difficult emotional fear? Mr. Delaware feared and anticipated that if he did not complete the second cycle of chemotherapy, then he too would not survive like his wife who was unable to complete chemotherapy. The past two years, he had a very difficult time because his wife had battled with breast cancer and had a terrible time undergoing chemotherapy. She could not tolerate chemotherapy and was only able to complete two cycles. He thought that was why she died a year ago. When he continued to regress on his wife, he became very anxious and fearful during chemotherapy. He reached a near breakdown point as he was having trouble breathing even while on canal oxygen. He finally realized and slowly came to understand the need to stay focused and try to take one day at a time. He also understood the need to avoid revisiting his wife's problems which caused pain and sadness. As he overcame his fear, he became more relaxed and strong. Despite several hospitalizations, including a placement of chest tube to help with drainage of lung fluid. He continued with months

of chemotherapy treatments. Even to the end, he was able to fulfill his life and enjoyed the best time with his daughter during the most difficult time in his life.

Words to live by

Buddhism:
"What you think you become."

Chapter 14
Distrust

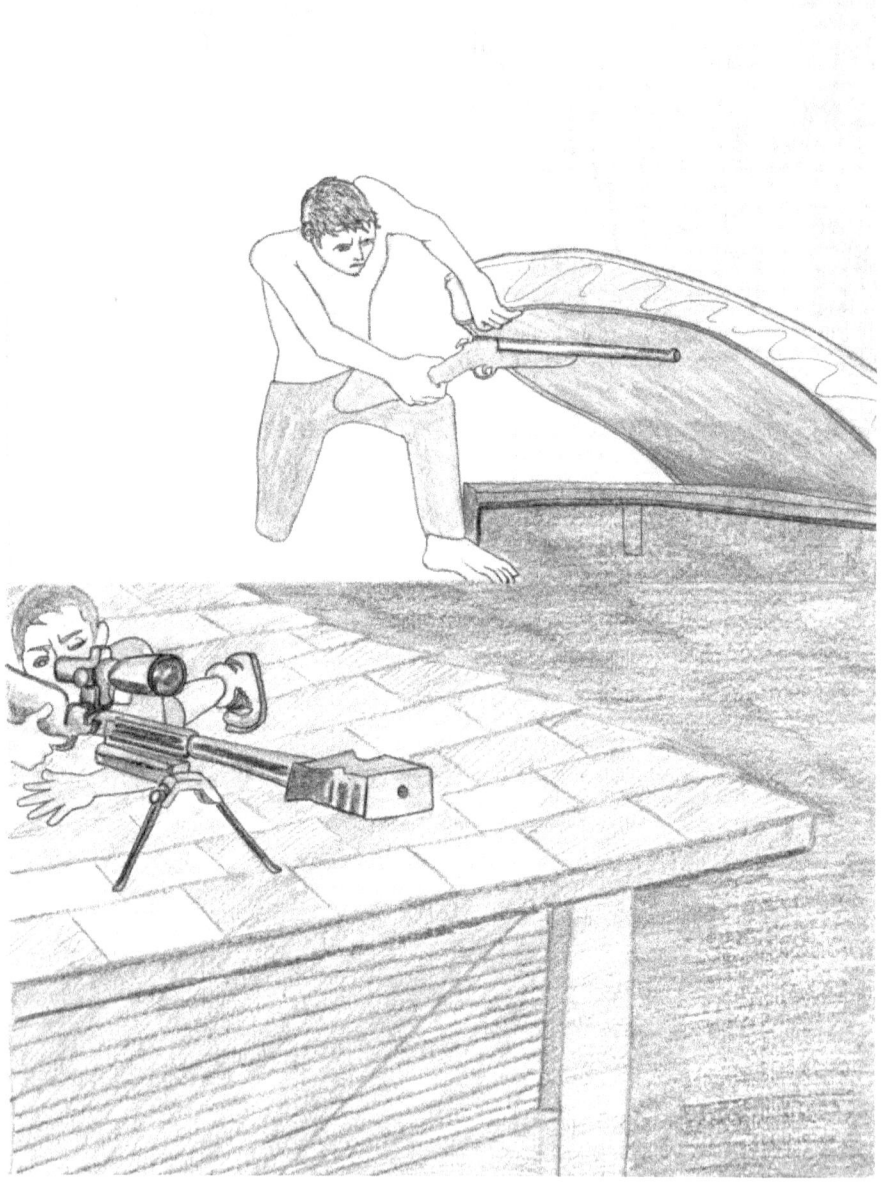

Mr. Georgia Jorge is a patient who had a long list of diseases including compensated cirrhosis of the liver and severe kidney failure. Mr. Georgia was a successful business man and cared very deeply for his mother. He resided with his mother after his wife passed away. He then married a lady who was about ten years younger. He bought a house right next to his previous house so that he could keep an eye on his mother. He had a very long history of abusing alcohol. His cancer was discovered after having about two months of rectal bleeding. After the work up, his cancer was diagnosed as stage II rectal cancer. Due to his complicated health situation, his cancer finding was presented to the Tumor Board for further evaluation.

The Tumor Board is a group of medical experts of surgeons, radiotherapists, oncologists and other specialists who meet to discuss what therapies are appropriate for a patient. Due to his poor liver and kidney function, they agreed to omit surgery at that time and he was sent to the oncology clinic to discuss treatment. Due to the stage of cancer, he qualified for chemo-radiation. After the completion of concurrent chemo-radiation therapy, his cancer continued to progress. Again, his case was presented to the Tumor Board which recommended that he receive supportive therapy due to his poor health. He again returned to the oncology clinic to discuss treatment options. He was previously seen by another oncology provider, but requested that his care be transferred to a different provider.

When I first met him and his wife, he was in a wheel chair, frail and looked as if he was in his nineties, rather than in his mid-sixties. He was so frail that his stature and the swelling of his abdomen from ascites was disproportionate. He was very upset with his previous oncologist thinking he did not provide enough help.

I explained that his failing kidney and liver disease was the reason he was offered supportive care rather than more chemotherapy or radiation. His anger took some time to resolve. As we continued with our **Fearlessness** session, he unveiled his tragic trapped life. He had been living in fear since returning from Vietnam over thirty years ago. He always kept two loaded rifles very nearby in the house. One rifle was placed under his pillow and another was kept in his mattress. These rifles had been those since his return from Vietnam. He described a horrific memory from when he was fighting in Vietnam. He fought alongside of what he called the "Tiger Scouts". Tiger Scouts were Vietnamese soldiers who took "point" for the American soldiers. During a firefight, he recalled vivid images of these Tiger Scouts getting killed, their blood and guts splattering all over his body. He also recalled he was captured, beaten up, and starved for days. He thought that he would die! Fortunately, he was able to escape with two little Vietnamese boys whom he befriended. The two boys ages nine and ten, had previously exchanged their rice for his canned food. The boys sneaked in one night, cut his wire cage, and helped him escape.

After returning from Vietnam, he continued to live in the **fearful past!**

He had worked in construction and purchased lots of equipment which he stored in his back yard. Some of his equipment had been stolen during the day and he expected the robbers to return at night to finish the job. On many occasions, he spent several nights on the roof of his house waiting for the robbers to return. I recalled asking him if he could see well enough in the dark to shoot accurately. He explained that he was a trained sniper and could shoot accurately over 190 meters. He had fired at the robbers in the past to scare them away; they had not yet returned.

To my amazement, following the first **Fearlessness** session, he returned using a walker. His wife related since that visit, he had been up and about every day, his appetite increased, and he was more relaxed. He even moved his rifles to the closet for the very first time, but wouldn't put them away for good. On that visit, he was informed that his cancer tumor was tested for a mutation and it was becoming a wild-type *K-ras* and would benefit from a new chemotherapy. He was reluctant to try the chemotherapy, fearing the side effects. He stated that he would continue seeing me monthly for support, but remained firm declining to try chemotherapy. Undoubtedly, he has **fear** of an **unknown future**.

For over six months, he remained strong, active and functional, occasionally requiring blood support due to his rectal bleeding. During his last few months, he was very happy and accomplished his goal of adding a pool to his house. As his wife later related, he had a very difficult time giving up the rifles, so they remained in the closet, but not under the pillow or mattress. During his wife's last visit; she stated that he had a peaceful passing.

Discussion 14:

How did Mr. Jorge live in fear since returning from Vietnam over thirty years ago? He always kept two loaded rifles very nearby in the house. One rifle was placed under his pillow and another was kept in his mattress.   As the "Tiger Scouts" were getting killed, their blood and guts splattered all over his body. Not only was he constantly flashing on these horrible images, he feared from the event when he was captured, beaten up and starved for days. Not only was he living in fear of his past, he feared of the unknown future. He spent several nights on the roof of his house waiting for the robbers to return. He was reluctant to try the chemotherapy, fearing the side effects. Although he was able to overcome his fear, he was unable to remain less fearful. However, during his last few months, he was very happy and accomplished his goal of adding a pool to his house. He moved his rifles to the closet for the very first time, but wouldn't put them away for good.

Words to live by

Buddhism:
"All that we are is the result of what we have thought."

GROUP IV
FEARFUL with RIGID/ATTACHED NOTION

Chapter 15
Obsess

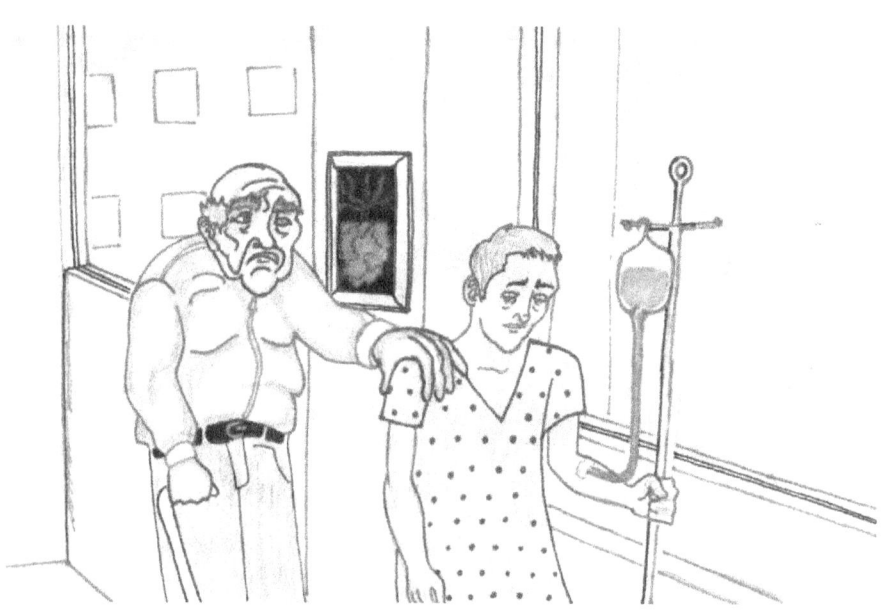

Mr. Brad Bentley is a patient who had a somewhat short list of medical diseases but unusual in that he also had a psychological disorder. Among other diseases, he was diagnosed with colon cancer. His colon cancer was found after having changes in his bowel movements involving abdominal pain.

Following a colonoscopy and CT scans, the biopsy showed that his cancer was from the colon and it was at an early stage. Therefore, surgery was offered and the cancer was removed. Although the disease was at its early stage, he still needed to be on adjuvant treatment.

For six months, his previous oncologists were unable to convince him to start the adjuvant chemotherapy. Hence, he was on observation. He later transferred to me to continue to be observed. On his very first visit, he appeared to be a very pleasant and calm patient, but he would speak of war events when under pressure. To maintain calm and to release his fear and stress, he would talk about the past, usually involving a historical event of the war. This was a part of his defence mechanism for his psychotic disorder. He did not have any family support. His only relative was an elderly great aunt who was living in a nursing home. He lived alone and was capable of caring for him, but had no means of transportation. He would arrange transportation through volunteer service or the clinic.

During each monthly visitation, he would explain that he did not have cancer. He was associating cancer with having pain, which he had before his surgery. He concluded that taking chemotherapy medication would give him cancer. After three months of persuasion during the **Fearlessness** sessions in hoping to resolve his fear, he agreed to give oral chemotherapy a try. He reasoned that intravenous chemotherapy was more toxic and that the newer pills would be less toxic. Also, he could take them at home. I was ecstatic and proud when he agreed to try it. But, he returned the oral chemotherapy in its original packaging at the very next visit. Again, he was unable to deviate from his fear and reasoning that cancer caused pain and that cancer medication (as a side effect) will cause cancer. For almost a year, he continued to feel and do well while on observation. As he was feeling and doing well, he missed several follow-up appointments.

One day he showed up at the clinic, without an appointment, and was referred to me immediately. When I asked why he came in that day, he said he got lucky. He was just taking an hour long walk around his neighbourhood. Suddenly a van appeared right next to him and the driver asked if he would like a ride to the clinic.

As it turned out, he came to see his primary doctor to request surgery, since he had pain in his stomach. Examination showed that his abdominal pain was caused by a mass that was palpable. As quickly as I could I convinced him that I needed to order the CT scans to see what was hurting him; he agreed. The CT scan confirmed that the cancer had returned and spread to his liver. His next visit, I arranged for a psychologist to be present when I offered him chemotherapy again. Neither the psychologist nor I were able to convince him to begin. The only treatment he wanted was to have the mass removed by surgery, since it was the only part of his body that caused pain. He was not a candidate for surgery due to the spread. He was referred for palliative care and, later to hospice care. He died shortly after. He was living with an extremely **rigid/rooted notion.**

Discussion 15:
What happened to Mr. Brad Bentley? For months, his previous oncologists were unable to convince him to start the adjuvant chemotherapy. He had reached an indestructible fear and it became part of his life. To avoid dealing with his **fear**, he spoke of war events. This was a part of his defence mechanism for his psychotic disorder. He associated his cancer with having pain, which he had before his surgery. He concluded that taking chemotherapy medication would give him cancer since he no longer had the pain. As his fear lessened, he agreed to give oral chemotherapy a try. He reasoned that intravenous chemotherapy was more toxic and that the newer pill form would be less toxic. But, he returned the oral chemotherapy in its original packaging at the very next visit. Again, he was unable to deviate from his fear and reasoning that cancer caused pain and that cancer medication (as side effect) will

cause cancer. In the end, the only treatment he wanted was to have the mass removed by surgery, since it was the only part of his body that caused pain. He was living with an extremely **rigid/rooted notion**.

Words to live by

Psalms 23:
The LORD is my shepherd; I shall not want.

Chapter 16
Rigid

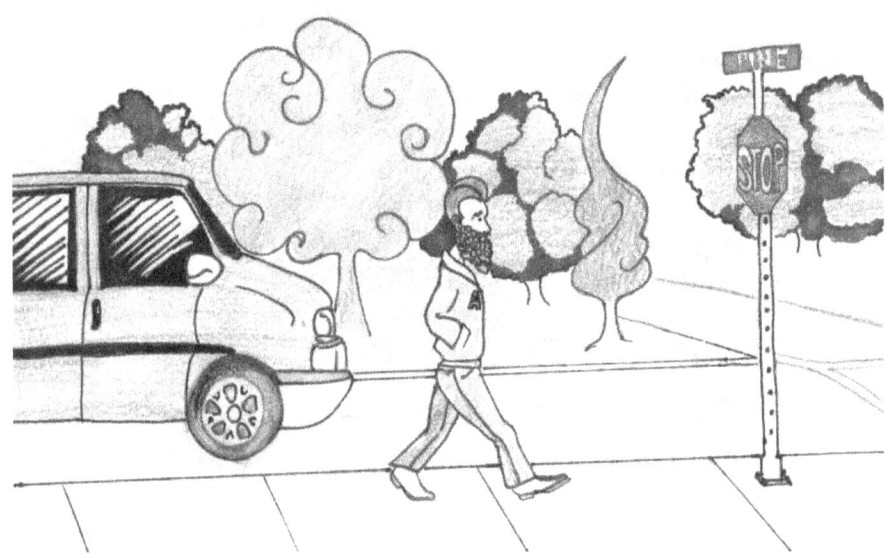

Mr. Art Arkansas is a patient who had esophageal cancer and a long history of alcohol abuse. For years, he had moved around the country living on his own. He remained single and did not have children.   He worked as a mechanic and enjoyed drinking alcohol every chance he had. He had been having difficulty swallowing for several months, but had little trouble when he drank. The difficult swallowing was usually with hard or with solid food. Then it quickly became difficult even with soft food. Then within a week, he was unable to swallow even liquid food or his alcohol. He quickly sought help and came to the emergency department. Due to severe weight loss and his inability to eat, he was admitted to the hospital. During the hospital stay, tests were obtained and a CT scan showed a mass in his upper mid chest. A biopsy was obtained and his cancer was discovered at a late stage (stage IV).

He quickly moved back to his parents for family support. He came to our clinic to begin treatment. He had been seeing another provider who started him on chemotherapy. He received only one cycle. Due to his displeasure with that provider, who he felt was too overbearing and belittling, he requested a transfer to another provider.

When he first saw me, he was very upset and expressed his anger regarding his previous provider. Due to much anger, he was offered **Fearlessness** to search for his fear to reduce his anger. During the discussion, it revealed that

Mr. Arkansas was very fixed on the idea that his esophageal cancer should be surgically removed. He envisioned a mechanical procedure for surgery that did not exist.   He insisted that the only problem or illness that he had was trouble swallowing. He held firm insisting over and over again that the surgeons needed to perform surgery to fix his problem.

After four weeks of much more persuasion and discussion, he agreed to try chemotherapy again. His elderly father, who came with him on a visit, was grateful that I was able to calm his son, and that I was able to convince him to resume treatment.   When he returned the following day to begin chemotherapy, the nurses noticed he was calm, pleasant and much more patient compared to his previous visits. He received almost two months of treatments, then missed several follow-up appointments. His elderly father later related that he was feeling better and able to eat, so he decided on his own not to come in. He was brought in by his father when he again had difficulty swallowing. He agreed to resume chemotherapy.

He took the treatments on and off, depending on the pain and the difficulty of swallowing. Shortly thereafter, he had much more difficulty swallowing and his disease progressed rapidly. He shredded weight; pounds a day. Again, he remained very fixed on his ideas of treatment. He insisted on surgery and refused further chemotherapy. He insisted that his cancer was so far advanced because surgery was not offered when he was first diagnosed. He was also upset that he was not offered surgery. Mr. Arkansas became more difficult, and his elderly father requested that his son receive assisted living. Caring for his son and his elderly wife had become overwhelming. Mr. Arkansas later was transferred to hospice care where he passed away. He was living with an extremely **rigid/rooted notion!**

Discussion 16:
Mr. Art Arkansas' story revealed another ultimate stage of fear. Mr. Arkansas was so fixed on the idea that his esophageal cancer should be surgically removed. He envisioned a mechanical procedure for surgery that did not exist and insisted. He insisted that the only problem or illness that he had was trouble swallowing. He held firm, insisting over and over again that the surgeons were to fix his problem. He was fixed on the idea of surgery as a solution to cure his cancer. His prolonged and chronic denial blended and prevented him from accepting the reality of having cancer and not simply a problem with digestion and difficulty swallowing. He remained in denial and fear.

Words to live by

Psalm 147:5:

Great is our Lord and mighty in power; his understanding has no limit.

UNDERSTANDING FEARLESSNESS

Let's turn back to the sixteen stories; there is a common thread that runs through these stories. The common thread is **fear**. **Fear** of the unknown future and past that result in ridged-rooted notions. The order of the groups corresponds to the severity of the problems. The problems vary from mild to very severe. Fixed thinking results in extreme **fear.** One has difficulty adjusting to new ideas or new places. In another words, the fixated mind is a mind that is very rooted which is the worst of all. Changes would be difficult if not impossible.

Though the **fear** can be of big or small, **fear** can cause **difficult emotional** experiences or **distress.** While **fear** can affect one individual in different ways, the more **significant** the **fear**, the more intense the experience will become. **Significance** or value of **fear** becomes of great importance because of personal attachment. Significance is the most important key factor in this process because it creates a deadlock of attachment. A deadlock between the significance and attachment creates emotional turmoil of **fear** leading to the destruction of health and eventually a process of disease.

Being able to adjust or having mental flexibility of acceptance is a tremendously important mechanism to overcome **fear.** A prolonged or a more complex attachment of **fear** creates a locked stage of **fear**. This deadlock stage leads to a **conflict** in the mind. Circumstances are what life does to an individual, but **fear** is what an individual does to oneself.

The process of the **emotional worries and stresses** resulting from **fear** starts with a **need**. But **need** becomes **important** or **significant** because of **wanting**. To obtain or fulfil this need, an exchange must take place. More often, this exchange is very difficult if not impossible to obtain... Not wanting a loved one to die...Not wanting to be diagnosed with cancer...Wanting to win the lottery's jackpot to pay off debts...Wanting to become rich and famous. Wanting to win...

Suffering becomes **depression** due to a continuation of failure to succeed in what is considered a significant need. Anticipation and hope to succeed will cause **anxiety** while waiting for it to happen. Repetition of anxiety and depression produces **fear**. In order to defeat fear, **anger** is often expressed. Both depressed and anxious people advocate impossibilities.

Frustration is a feeling of dissatisfaction, often accompanied by anxiety or depression, resulting from unfulfilled needs or unresolved problems. Therefore, the more wanting is involved, the more suffering (distress) results from frustration.

There are individuals who are currently living in the present time, but are unable to be uprooted from their **fearful** past. Basically, they are living in the past but in the present time. They are here, but really they are not. On the other hand, there are many individuals who are living in **fear**, worrying about their next hour or future. Again, they are there and not really here. One can see that it is difficult to remove a built in wall unit or a deeply rooted tree with ease and without killing it. This process is difficult. The wall unit is torn apart and the tree will die if it is not done properly.

CONCLUSION

Changes produce emotional experiences or distress. **Ideal** and **real** are two different concepts, but they have a major effect on **fear**. Ideal is a state of perfection where everything is as you wish. There is no fear in the **ideal** state. **Real** is a state of constant changes and is imperfect. In turn, the **real** will create **fear**-Not wanting a loved one to die; being diagnosed with a terminal disease like cancer; becoming disabled from a severe accident; becoming dependence and having less physical strength and youth due to aging; having less income from retirement, jobless, or ending a relationship with divorce. Other **real** experiences are those of comfort needs such as moving away from familiar home, or as simple as just starting school for children can also form **fear**. The difficult **emotional experiences or distress** from undergoing these changes produce pain, hurt, suffering, trouble, hardship, and at times vindictiveness all of which can create **fear**.

Fearlessness was designed initially to help cancer patients deal with the difficult emotional experiences that they go through from the time they are diagnosed with cancer. As a result, it helped cancer patients as well as their friends and family members calm their fright, bring fulfillment to their lives and often, delay and free them from their disease.

To successfully overcome **fear**, one must be able to **adapt and accept** the changes. Circumstances are what life does to an individual, but **fear** is what the individual does to oneself.

I am not a philosopher or a preacher, but for many decades great philosophers as well as religious practitioners have tried to explain this process of **Fearlessness** in so many ways and forms. The only person in charge of your life is you! You have the power of closure from your past and to control your future. If you remain in the past or look too far into the future, your reality will be stolen away. That is a very dangerous place to be. For the past had moved on; and the future will change. The future can only be prepared for, but be careful!! The anticipation of waiting for the next hour will drain your wealth of health!

Glossary

Erythrocytosis: an abnormally high level of hematocrit and hemoglobin

Gaisbock's disease: hypovolemia or tress erythrocytosis. There are no known treatment guidelines for Gaisbock's syndrome, other than to drink more water to expand the vascular volume

Hemachromatosis: a disorder of too much iron accumulation in the body which can lead to organ toxicity.

Idiopathic/immune thrombocytopenia purpura (ITP): a disease that can cause an increased risk of bleeding

Leukocytosis: an elevation of white blood counts commonly found during the infection process which can be a form of leukemia

Multiple myeloma: a plasma cell cancer that grows in the bone

Myelodysplasic syndrome (MDS): a bone marrow and blood disease that can be either in a mild or severe form of preleukemia. The milder form can be easily managed, but the severe form can progress and become a full blown leukemia. Estimates indicate that about 10 % of the patients with MDS will progress to leukemia. Patients with this form of life-threatening MDS, have a very short time to live. Medical experts do not know the cause of the changes to the bone marrow.

Pancytopenia: a reduction of blood cells that can cause serious life-threatening illnesses.

Special Thanks To:

Charles W.
Dennis C.
Frederick S.
Lee E.
Raymond G.

For further information, please visit website:
choosefearlessness.com

A production of fearlessness
Management & Consultant.